THE
CLINICAL
RESEARCH
HANDBOOK

A Practical Guide to Designing, Conducting, and Publishing Clinical Research

THE CLINICAL RESEARCH HANDBOOK

A Practical Guide to Designing, Conducting, and Publishing Clinical Research

Mohammad Faizan Khan
Indiana University, USA

Nolan J Brown
University of California Irvine, USA

Julian Gendreau
Johns Hopkins University, USA

Ronald Sahyouni
University of California San Diego, USA

Aaron Cohen-Gadol
University of Southern California, USA

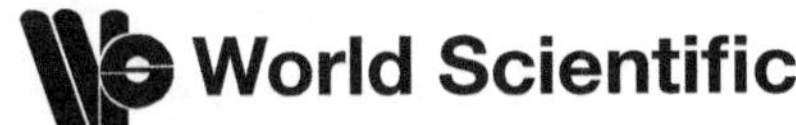

NEW JERSEY · LONDON · SINGAPORE · BEIJING · SHANGHAI · TAIPEI · CHENNAI

Published by

World Scientific Publishing Co. Pte. Ltd.

5 Toh Tuck Link, Singapore 596224

USA office: 27 Warren Street, Suite 401-402, Hackensack, NJ 07601

UK office: 57 Shelton Street, Covent Garden, London WC2H 9HE

British Library Cataloguing-in-Publication Data
A catalogue record for this book is available from the British Library.

THE CLINICAL RESEARCH HANDBOOK
A Practical Guide to Designing, Conducting and Publishing Clinical Research

ISBN 978-981-98-1459-6 (hardcover)
ISBN 978-981-98-1572-2 (paperback)
ISBN 978-981-98-1460-2 (ebook for institutions)
ISBN 978-981-98-1461-9 (ebook for individuals)

For any available supplementary material, please visit
https://www.worldscientific.com/worldscibooks/10.1142/14351#t=suppl

Preface

Through clinical research, field-changing ideas are formulated, tested, and ultimately translated into clinical practice with the goal of improving healthcare for generations to come. In this regard, an individual can test and discover knowledge that has never been brought to fruition in the present medical community, and the researcher can be the first to see this information first-hand.

From a practical perspective, there is a need for medical students, both in the United States, and internationally, to be exposed to clinical research in their medical education. In the United States, many students are encouraged to perform research in medical school for the overall advancement of the field and also to become competitive for the medical residency match process. The latter point has become even more important over the past two years as Step 1 has recently become pass/fail, and thus, many students are turning to research to become competitive candidates in their field of interest.

However, in the clinical environment, academic mentors are often busy and, in some medical schools, difficult to find. Therefore, students in these situations need a written resource that describes how to perform research for junior medical professionals. Internationally, some medical students may have difficulties finding mentors to guide them to perform effective clinical research. Therefore, in *A Practical Guide to Clinical Research: For Medical Students and Other Junior Healthcare Professionals*, the authors attempt to provide a concise and effective reading that allows individuals to gain introductory knowledge in performing clinical research. We completely describe the process of research by describing how to formulate ideas, act upon those ideas, and submit these ideas as publishable manuscripts to journals.

Specifically, we cover many key concepts, such as reading relevant peer-reviewed literature, formulating novel hypotheses, describing the basic fundamentals of formatting, writing a manuscript, and different types of data sources, such as institutional datasets and many national databases that are now offered to clinicians. We describe how to take this data and perform statistical analysis using the prominent packages using the RStudio program, and we additionally provide basic source code for medical students in each chapter. Finally, we discuss the creation of online predictive calculators, which are becoming even more common in literature today.

Where possible, we take all opportunities to explain these subjects in non-technical and easy-to-understand terms, and each chapter is designed to be read as a unique individual reading in an effort to save time for the reader. Since this is primarily aimed at individuals who are junior in their careers, we aim to make this reading as low of a cost as possible. Using our proposed book, medical students will be able to go from formulating ideas to getting their manuscripts accepted by using all of the information provided here.

Contents

Part I
Getting Started

1 Selecting Meaningful Research Projects for Real-World Impact

Introduction

Research is a powerful force for change. Whether addressing global healthcare disparities, improving local community services, advancing technology, or exploring the frontiers of science, well-chosen research projects can solve practical problems and expand our understanding of the world. However, identifying the "right" question is often the hardest — and most critical — step in this journey.

This chapter provides a detailed, step-by-step guide to help you navigate the process of selecting a research project that aligns with your passions, meets pressing societal needs, and stands up to rigorous scrutiny. We will explore how to:

- Integrate personal inspiration with the broader community or societal priorities
- Conduct a thorough review of existing literature to identify genuine gaps
- Use established frameworks to formulate a clear and answerable question
- Balance ambitious ideas with feasible plans
- Build a long-term research trajectory that can shape your career or future endeavors.

By the end, you should be equipped with practical strategies for crafting research questions that matter — not only to you but also to the communities and fields you hope to serve.

Aligning Your Interests with Broader Needs

Finding Personal Inspiration

Intrinsic motivation fuels persistence. Research projects are seldom straightforward; they often involve setbacks, complex logistics, and lengthy timelines. A meaningful personal connection to the topic helps sustain energy and focus when challenges arise. The following is a list of strategies for personal discovery:

- **Reflect on personal or professional experiences**
  - Think of moments where you witnessed a problem firsthand — perhaps in a clinic, a workplace, or a community program. These "on-the-ground" experiences can illuminate real, unmet needs.
- **Engage in constant exploration**
  - Attend webinars, guest lectures, or community forums. Keep a notepad or digital file of interesting ideas and questions you encounter.
- **Leverage curiosity**
  - Ask "Why?" whenever you see a phenomenon that interests you, even if it seems tangential. Some of the most groundbreaking research questions arise from everyday observations.

A practical example of using this framework would be a student who watched a family member struggle with side effects from chemotherapy and may feel driven to explore ways to reduce toxicity.

This personal connection can guide the student toward researching novel drug-delivery systems or supportive care interventions.

Identifying Urgent Issues

While personal passion is vital, connecting that passion to a real-world need amplifies the potential impact. Whether your area is medical research, education, business, environmental science, or technology, pinpointing urgent and unsolved problems increases the relevance — and often the support and funding — of your project. The following is a list of strategies that can be utilized for identifying urgent issues:

- **Consult public health and policy reports**
  - o Organizations like the World Health Organization (WHO), the United Nations (UN), or national institutes publish regular reports highlighting pressing global or local issues (e.g., the burden of non-communicable diseases and environmental pollution hotspots).
- **Engage with local communities or end users**
  - o Community groups, patient advocacy organizations, industry roundtables, or school boards can articulate their most pressing challenges and help shape your research trajectory.
- **Monitor emerging trends**
  - o Be alert to new technologies, shifting demographics, or policy changes that might create gaps or opportunities (e.g., the rise of telehealth, aging populations, or climate change impacts on agriculture).

A practical example of using this framework would be a public health advocate who notices that diabetes prevalence is skyrocketing in low-income areas. Identifying this as an urgent health disparity can spur research into cost-effective lifestyle interventions, mobile health apps for medication reminders, or policy changes that incentivize healthier food options.

Balancing Personal Passion with External Impetus

A project at the intersection of personal interest and broader needs is most likely to sustain momentum and secure stakeholder buy-in. This balance is crucial for ensuring both longevity and wider applicability. To map your interests with existing gaps, create a simple two-column chart listing: (a) personal research interests and (b) pressing societal or field-specific problems. Look for overlaps or synergy. Additionally, seeking feedback is important as sometimes, mentors, peers, or professionals with experience in a particular domain can shed light on which emerging problems most urgently need attention — and which are the most feasible.

Reviewing What's Already Known

When developing an idea, you can review what is already discovered on the topic by using two primary data sources. This would include both systematic reviews and scoping (narrative) reviews. Before committing to a research direction, it is essential to understand the state of current knowledge. By doing so, you avoid duplicating existing work and identify potential areas where your contribution could be unique.

- **Systematic reviews**
  - Definition: A highly structured approach (often guided by PRISMA (Preferred Reporting Items for Systematic Review and Meta-Analyses)) that specifies search criteria, databases used, and strict inclusion/exclusion rules.

- o Benefits: Delivers rigorous, quantitative summaries (e.g., meta-analyses) and identifies data-driven consensus or the lack thereof.
  - o Challenges: Tends to be time-consuming and is best suited when your research question is already quite focused.
- **Scoping or narrative reviews**
  - o Definition: Broader, more exploratory overviews that gather information on a wide range of sources without rigid protocols.
  - o Benefits: Ideal if you are still refining your question or seeking a broad conceptual understanding of the field.
  - o Challenges: May not provide the precise effect sizes or strict quality assessments that systematic reviews offer.

Spotting Knowledge Gaps

Real innovation occurs when researchers address what has not been resolved or explored. Gaps can include contradictory findings, unexplored populations, or novel research methods that have not yet been applied to a known problem. There are several optimal ways to identify gaps in current knowledge:

- **Look for contradictions**
  - o Are there studies that show opposite results under seemingly similar conditions? This discrepancy may point to methodological weaknesses or unrecognized confounders.
- **Focus on special populations**
  - o Some demographics (e.g., older adults, rural communities, underrepresented minorities) might be underrepresented in large studies, even if they bear a high burden of disease.

- **Embrace interdisciplinary insights**
  - Check if theories or methods from another field (e.g., data science, behavioral economics, or engineering) could be applied to your domain in a novel way.
  - Practical example

An example of contradictory findings would be if Study A finds a strong correlation between a certain diet and reduced cardiovascular risk, while Study B finds no such correlation. Investigating the differences in population genetics, dietary measurement methods, or confounding factors (like exercise habits) can open an exciting line of research.

Triangulating from Multiple Literatures

Sometimes, meaningful insights emerge only after synthesizing information from different sources or disciplines. Public health challenges often intersect with economics, psychology, or technological innovations. These can be discovered using interdisciplinary databases such as broad academic search engines (e.g., Google Scholar, Scopus) and domain-specific repositories (e.g., IEEE Xplore for engineering, PsycINFO for psychology) to gather diverse perspectives. It can also take the form of expert consultations with professionals from different fields that can guide you toward lesser-known but potentially relevant literature.

Turning Your Interests into Answerable Questions

Using the FINER Criteria

FINER (Feasible, Interesting, Novel, Ethical, Relevant) ensures your project is practical, intellectually stimulating, socially (or scientifically) beneficial, and responsibly conducted.

- <u>F</u>easible
  - o Do you have access to participants, data, lab equipment, or necessary software tools?
  - o Is your timeline realistic given institutional or personal deadlines?
- <u>I</u>nteresting
  - o Will you remain motivated throughout the project's duration?
  - o Does the question pique the curiosity of potential collaborators or broader audiences?
- <u>N</u>ovel
  - o Are you genuinely adding fresh insight or using a new method?
  - o Even if the topic is well-studied, a different approach or population might uncover new facets.
- <u>E</u>thical
  - o Are risks to participants minimized, and have you planned robust informed consent processes?
  - o Have you addressed privacy concerns if using sensitive data (e.g., health records)?
- <u>R</u>elevant
  - o Who benefits if you answer this question — patients, policymakers, educators, or industry stakeholders?
  - o Could results influence guidelines, best practices, or future research directions?

Framing with PICO (and Other Variations)

PICO (Population, Intervention, Comparator, Outcome) brings clarity by defining the "who," "what," and "how" of your research question. This structure makes your objectives explicit and your design more rigorous.

- <u>P</u>opulation: Describe demographics or relevant characteristics (e.g., children aged 6–10 with ADHD, software users in large corporations, etc.).
- <u>I</u>ntervention: Identify the variable or program being introduced or studied (e.g., a new medication, a behavioral strategy, a software update).
- <u>C</u>omparator: Decide on the baseline or control condition (e.g., placebo, previous software version, standard practice).
- <u>O</u>utcome: Clarify what success or measurement of interest looks like (e.g., improvement in symptoms, user satisfaction, cost reduction).

Other variants of this framework are the PICOT acronym, which adds a timeframe (e.g., 6-month follow-up), the SPICE acronym (<u>S</u>etting, <u>P</u>erspective, <u>I</u>ntervention, <u>C</u>omparison, <u>E</u>valuation), often used in social sciences or qualitative contexts, and the PICOS acronym (<u>P</u>opulation, <u>I</u>ntervention, <u>C</u>omparator, <u>O</u>utcome, <u>S</u>tudy design), which is particularly helpful for structuring systematic reviews. Additional frameworks can also be included in other fields such as SMART Goals being <u>S</u>pecific, <u>M</u>easurable, <u>A</u>chievable, <u>R</u>elevant, and <u>T</u>ime-bound — useful in project management or implementation science. Additionally, logic models are often used in community-based or public health research to link inputs, activities, outputs, and outcomes, clarifying how your intervention leads to change.

Balancing Ambition with Practical Realities

Assessing Resource Feasibility

Even the most brilliant idea can flounder if you lack critical resources (e.g., funding, lab equipment, software expertise, or participant access). This can be performed by looking through your inventory for available resources. This would include writing down everything at your disposal, from budget lines and mentorship to specialized lab facilities. Cultivating partnerships is also crucial. If you need advanced statistical methods, consider collaborating with a data science department or a research consultancy. Plan your timeline carefully by mapping out your project's stages — literature review, data collection, analysis, and manuscript writing — and gauge each phase's duration. Be realistic and build in buffers.

Weighing Risk vs. Reward

Cutting-edge research can yield high-impact results but also carries more uncertainty (e.g., untested methods, regulatory hurdles). Conversely, a safer project might guarantee some publishable findings but may not push the envelope. Strategies for this can include the use of pilot studies, or a small-scale test can reveal feasibility issues, unexpected costs, or design flaws without jeopardizing your entire plan. Develop contingency plans, which outline alternative paths if you encounter major obstacles (e.g., if participant recruitment is slower than expected). Finally, consider creating adaptive designs that let you modify aspects of the study as interim results come in.

Timelines, Synergy, and Initial Wins

Progress milestones help keep you motivated and demonstrate to funders or supervisors that the project is on track. During this process, set short-, medium-, and long-term goals. For instance, aim to complete the literature review within two months, pilot data collection within six months, and final data analysis by the end of the year. Celebrate small successes, whether it is finishing a pilot or securing ethics approval — acknowledging milestones helps maintain momentum. Stay flexible. Timelines are guidelines, not rigid constraints. Adjust as new data or obstacles emerge.

Crafting a Long-Term Research Path

Finding and Building Your Research Niche

Over time, focusing on a particular area of interest helps you establish expertise and recognition. This can lead to sustained funding, invitations to collaborate, and leadership roles.

- **Choose a focal point**
  - You might center on a disease (e.g., Type 2 diabetes), a technique (e.g., genetic sequencing), or a theoretical framework (e.g., behavioral economics in education).
- **Develop depth and breadth**
  - Depth: Continuously update your knowledge in your niche.
  - Breadth: Look for interdisciplinary opportunities — maybe combining microbiology with artificial intelligence (AI) or public health with environmental science.
- **Share your work widely**
  - Publish in journals, present at conferences, or write for public-facing platforms. Visibility fuels recognition.

Cultivating Collaborations and Mentorships

Complex problems often require multidisciplinary expertise. Collaborations can expand your capabilities, open new perspectives, and increase the likelihood of impactful findings.

Attend conferences and seminars, or join academic social networks (e.g., ResearchGate, LinkedIn groups). In academia, forming a mentorship group with experts from different fields can guide you on both scientific and career matters. Offer your own expertise or resources in return — true collaborations are mutual, not one-sided.

Ethics, Regulations, and Funding

Upholding Ethical and Regulatory Standards

Whether working with human participants, sensitive data, or environmental interventions, ethical guidelines ensure safety, rights, and transparency.

- **Informed consent**
  - o Participants should understand the study's purpose, procedures, potential risks, and benefits.
- **Privacy and confidentiality**
  - o Adhere to relevant data protection laws (e.g., HIPAA, GDPR) and anonymize sensitive information where possible.
- **Conflict of interest**
  - o Disclose any financial or professional relationships that might influence your research design or results interpretation.
- **Regulatory compliance**
  - o Check if you need approvals from ethics committees, institutional review boards (IRBs), or governmental bodies, especially for clinical or environmental studies.

Planning for Dissemination

Research has limited value if it remains locked in a drawer or behind paywalls. Effective dissemination ensures that relevant stakeholders — clinicians, policymakers, educators, and communities — can learn from your findings. These dissemination outlets can include academic journals and conferences, which are standard for scholarly communities, offering peer review and professional networking. Policy briefs are summaries geared toward legislators or agencies that can use evidence for decision-making. Community presentations and workshops are ideal for engaging non-academic audiences, including local groups or patient advocates. Open access repositories are great for archiving your work in public repositories (e.g., arXiv, institutional repositories), which broadens its reach.

Embracing an Iterative Process

No research plan is perfect from the start. Flexibility and openness to feedback can dramatically improve your study's quality. You can embrace an iterative process by:

- **Early presentations**
  - Present your idea at lab meetings, local conferences, or online forums to gather multiple perspectives.
- **Seek mentorship and peer reviews**
  - Constructive critiques can reveal hidden assumptions, suggest new methods, or point out oversights.
- **Stay informed on developments**
  - Keep an eye out for new studies or technologies that might affect your research design or interpretation.

Pilot Studies and "Test Runs"

Pilot work can save time and resources by catching obstacles early, such as unworkable methods, recruitment issues, or unexpected confounders.

- **Feasibility pilots**
  - Recruit a small cohort to test procedures, measurements, or interventions.
- **Prototype testing**
  - In tech or product design, trial runs with limited functions can expose user experience problems.
- **Interim analysis in clinical or community trials**
  - Evaluate partial data to confirm assumptions about effect sizes, dropout rates, or other factors.

Illustrative Examples

Chronic Pain Management

Scenario: You observe many chronic pain patients relying heavily on medication with limited access to non-pharmacological interventions.

Literature findings: Some small trials suggest mindfulness-based therapies can help, but larger studies with consistent measures are lacking.

Research question: "Does combining mindfulness-based stress reduction with standard physical therapy improve pain outcomes more than physical therapy alone for adults with chronic low back pain?"

Potential impact: If results show improvement, this approach could be integrated into standard care, potentially reducing opioid dependence.

Table 1.1.   PICO Breakdown for the Chronic Pain Management Scenario

Framework	Breakdown
Population	Adults (age 18+) with chronic low back pain.
Intervention	Eight-week mindfulness program in addition to physiotherapy (PT).
Comparator	PT alone.
Outcome	Self-reported pain scales, function tests, and medication usage.

Telemedicine in Rural Communities

Scenario: Public health data reveal high travel costs and limited specialist access in remote areas, contributing to poor disease management.

Literature findings: Telemedicine works in some settings, but cost-effectiveness and patient satisfaction data vary widely.

Research question: "In rural populations with diabetes, does telemedicine-based specialist consultation reduce healthcare costs and improve glycemic control compared to standard in-person care?"

Potential impact: Findings could guide resource allocation and policy decisions on reimbursing telehealth solutions.

Table 1.2.   PICO Breakdown for Telemedicine in the Rural Communities Scenario

Framework	Breakdown
Population	Rural diabetes patients with limited local specialist services.
Intervention	Telemedicine visits plus remote monitoring.
Comparator	Traditional in-person care.
Outcome	Change in HbA1c levels, total healthcare costs, patient satisfaction surveys.

Machine Learning for Environmental Monitoring

Scenario: Concern grows about water contamination in urban fringe areas near industrial zones.

Literature findings: Multiple small-scale studies examine local pollutants, but predictive models are often simplistic or outdated.

Research question: "Can a novel machine learning model more accurately predict regional water contamination risks than standard regression-based methods?"

Potential impact: Early detection of at-risk regions could prompt timely corrective measures, reducing health risks and environmental damage.

Table 1.3.　PICO Breakdown for the Machine Learning for Environmental Monitoring Scenario

Framework	Breakdown
Population	Geographic areas with known industrial runoff.
Intervention	Machine learning approach using satellite data and historical contamination reports.
Comparator	Traditional regression-based predictions used by local authorities.
Outcome	Prediction accuracy (e.g., F1 score), cost of false positives/negatives for water safety interventions.

Conclusion

Selecting a meaningful research project is a multi-layered process that merges personal inspiration with systematic inquiry. Let your personal experiences fuel your creativity, but validate their significance through data, policy priorities, or community input.

Systematic or scoping reviews ensure you build on existing knowledge and illuminate genuine gaps. Frameworks like FINER and PICO create clarity, guide your study design, and enhance rigor. Thoughtful resource planning, realistic timelines, and pilot studies help you scale your project effectively. Sustaining a focused niche, cultivating mentorship, and consistently publishing or presenting can establish you as an expert in your domain. Remaining flexible, being open to feedback and being committed to the highest ethical standards underpins trustworthy and beneficial research outcomes.

Ultimately, a well-conceived research project does more than contribute to academic discourse — it can shape clinical practice, inform public policy, empower communities, and foster innovations that transform lives. By following the principles laid out in this chapter, you set yourself on a path to produce work that is not only publishable but also truly impactful.

Additional Recommended Readings

- Farrugia P, Petrisor BA, Farrokhyar F, *et al*. Research questions, hypotheses and objectives. *Canadian Journal of Surgery*. 2010; **53**(4): 278–281.
- Greenhalgh T. *How to Read a Paper: The Basics of Evidence-Based Medicine*. 6th ed. London: BMJ Books; 2019.
- Guyatt G, Rennie D, Meade MO, *et al*. *Users' Guides to the Medical Literature: Essentials of Evidence-Based Clinical Practice*. 3rd ed. New York: McGraw-Hill Education; 2015.
- Hulley SB, Cummings SR, Browner WS, *et al*. *Designing Clinical Research*. 4th ed. Philadelphia: Lippincott Williams & Wilkins; 2013.
- Moher D, Liberati A, Tetzlaff J, *et al*. The PRISMA Group. Preferred reporting items for systematic reviews and meta-analyses: The PRISMA statement. *PLOS Medicine*. 2009; **6**(7): e1000097.

Chapter **2** Formulating Ideas

Research is critical for innovating the field of medicine. A medical student's aspirations to pursue research may stem from multiple different motivations. Students may wish to pursue research to become immersed in their particular field of interest, students may pursue research to bolster their CVs for job applications, and students may also be interested in making the field better for generations to come. Others may simply be required to perform clinical research as a result of one's job requirements.

What is Research? Research in a Nutshell

As a broad overview, medical research is a process where an investigator develops a scientific hypothesis that is rigorously tested using very strictly described guidelines. It can be described as the Scientific method, which consists of seven steps (Fig. 2.1).

Notice that all the steps of the scientific method are organized as a revolving circle and are not a beginning or an end. The scientific process is a continually ongoing concept that leads to the advancement of present-day healthcare systems. We will go into the details on how to practically implement all of these stages of the scientific method with the knowledge contained in the future chapters, but this figure is a good overview.

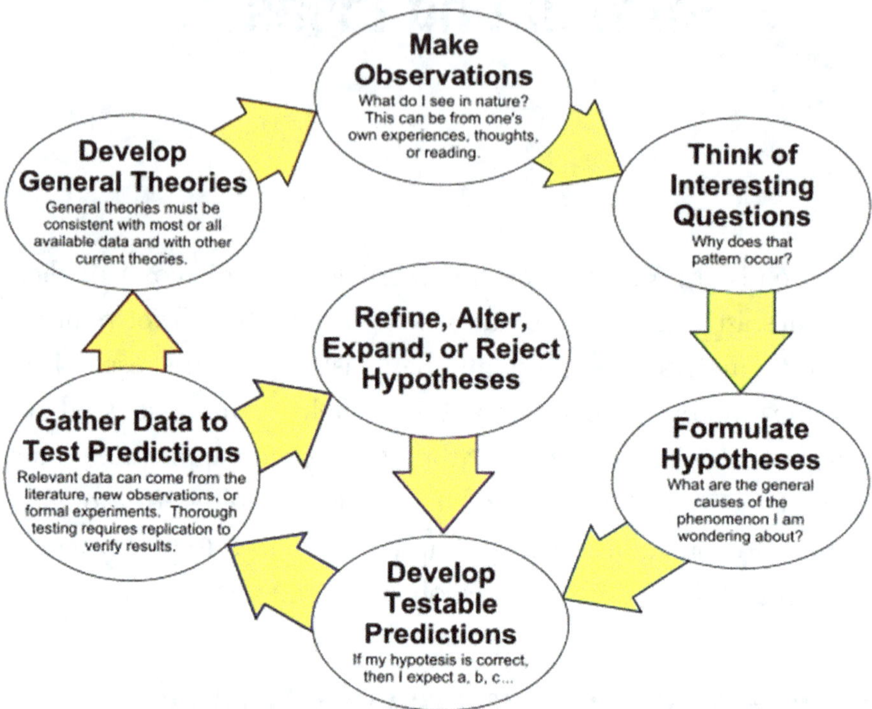

Fig. 2.1.   The Scientific Method as an Ongoing Process.[1]

Formulating Novel Ideas/Hypotheses

How does a junior individual develop an idea of one's own? There are two options for developing ideas as a junior scientist. The first and the most common option is to inherit or perform studies associated with your primary mentor. This is what most students will do during medical school or any professional school. The mentor has more knowledge in the field than the junior mentee, and the mentor knows the pertinent questions to ask and answer at that particular time in the field. Questions are always changing as the field continues to innovate; therefore, it is imperative that you have the right questions to ask and at the right time. Therefore, this is generally the best way to formulate research questions as a junior scientist.

Other individuals will be performing research questions that are pertinent to their particular job/industry. For example, if one is employed in the pharmaceutical industry, they will obviously be performing research ideas congruent to industry-specified goals. These tasks are often set by lead administrators with very rigid guidelines. Sometimes, they will even be performing studies with parameters that are specifically annotated by the company to prove feasibility or superior product. In these cases, it is easy to formulate an idea as someone has essentially completed this process for you.

But what if you are a medical student attempting to become involved in a field where you have no department at your school? What if you are a junior scientist who currently does not have a mentor in your field but you wish to produce research? First, one of the best things to do would be to find a mentor. Mentorship is key in medicine and crucial for advancement in one's career. However, what if you do not have a mentor currently and need to formulate ideas by yourself? We will discuss that as well.

Formulating Ideas Solo as a Junior Researcher

One key aspect of formulating ideas yourself would be to review journals in your field. This can be performed with a quick online search. For example, a medical student interested in endocrinology should attempt to find the top endocrinology journals available. This can be easily compared using a journal's impact factors.

A journal's impact factor is how many times a particular article was cited over one year, with the higher impact factor denoting more influential journals. In 2023, the *New England Journal of Medicine* was rated with an impact factor of 96.2,[2] which is very high. It is actually the highest in the journals in the field of medicine. On the other end of the spectrum, journals can have an impact factor of one or an average of one citation per year per article included in the journal. Some journals that are new or not widely supported and cited do not even have impact factors. When formulating ideas, you want to be reading from the highest impact factor journals of your field.

Finding the top impact factor journals in your field can be easily performed with online searches and websites. For example, the SJR Scimago Journal & Country Rank is a valuable website that provides impact factors for each field.[3] Google Scholar can also be used to find top journals by the h5-index, which is somewhat different than the impact factors. The h5-index is the number of articles published in the last five years that have a high number of citations. For example, if a journal has six articles published in the last five years that have six citations, then the journal has an h5-index of six. If a journal has 100 articles published in the last five years that are cited 100 times, then the h5-index is 100.

In general, to gather new ideas, you want to be current on the top journals in your field with high-impact factors and h5-indexes. From this, keeping current with the recent literature is critical. What questions are being answered in recently published studies? Do the studies currently published lead to new avenues of investigation? Some studies specifically mention future research opportunities at the end of their manuscripts. Is there an opportunity to use an article's technique of investigating another disease of interest? Are you able to transfer this type of investigation to the disease you would like to study? When you read many different articles in the literature, you will find that many of the articles have the same investigational processes. For example, there are many investigations using the Surveillance, Epidemiology, and End Results database (SEER) and the National Cancer Database

(NCD). Of these studies, there are typically different methods of investigation, such as investigating overall survival, surgical recommendations, disparities in access to care, etc. It can be helpful to find one of these methodologies in the current literature and apply it to new diseases that have not already been published or well described.

If you believe you have an idea, it is best to first perform a search on PubMed to see if it has been done previously. If you begin a study and attempt to publish a study that is already in PubMed or very similar to a study in PubMed, your chances of getting it accepted into a good journal significantly and drastically go down. Publishing duplicate studies is not advised, as it is difficult to publish, and it clutters the literature with redundant articles. Occasionally, it is acceptable to publish an update on studies with new data, but this can be difficult and is typically reserved for prior high-impact studies that have had a lot of updates in the medical outcomes since the prior published data.

In addition to searching the currently published literature, another avenue of finding ideas is to attend conferences in the field you wish to pursue. Many fields of medicine host both national and local conferences that are free of charge for medical students. Attending these is paramount, as it is great for networking and additionally for being in touch with the most recent advancements. The benefit of conferences is that many of the late and breaking studies are not fully ready to be published in journals yet but can be found being presented at conferences.

Many investigators first describe study findings at a conference, get feedback, and then publish the manuscript after attending the conference with their ideas. This was actually the way the process was intended to be originally. Conferences were attended before manuscript publication to receive feedback before publishing a final manuscript. Therefore, as a student, this would be a method for being up to date on the most recent research. At the conference, visit different posters. Ask people to describe their research — most investigators are looking forward to people asking about their work and forming collaborations with other individuals at the conference. It never hurts to simply ask someone to explain his or her poster. Additionally, attend oral presentations of interest. Hearing these presentations will give you new and up-to-date ideas.

One additional method of formulating ideas may seem simple but is often overlooked by students. Attending institutional grand rounds or weekly education conferences is key to getting baseline knowledge. Oftentimes, a unique patient will be admitted, which could be a case report. Attending clinics with your desired specialty is crucial to gaining a strong baseline that is required to innovate your field.

Final Deliverables

First, once you have preliminary data from your study, you would generally submit your work to a local or national conference. It is generally accepted that you can submit your work to both a local and national conference. However, it would not be generally accepted to submit your work to multiple national conferences. For example, if you have a new study with significant findings, it is not advisable to submit your work to five national conferences in the United States. Generally, most national conferences even have a disclaimer when submitting your abstract and work that specifically states this concept.

Once submitted to a conference, you are expected to travel to the conference and present your work for the purpose of obtaining feedback. The types of presentations can vary; however, these are generally in some form of electronic poster, print poster, short oral presentation, and full presentation.

Electronic posters are electronic Powerpoint slides that are displayed on a revolving screen at the conference and are the least desired, generally speaking. A print poster means the poster is up during the entire conference for people to view; however, there will be a set timeframe (a couple of hours usually), where individuals will stand next to their poster and give a two-minute presentation for conference attendees to ask questions. Sometimes, during this process, there is an additional poster competition, and then your two-minute speech is rated against your peers. The next two types of presentations are oral presentations where you would deliver a podium talk to conference attendees. The short presentation is generally <15 minutes in length and with a small room of people interested in that subspecialty. However, the full oral presentation can last up to 30 minutes and may involve the entire conference at a general meeting of the convention during a plenary session. Obviously, the latter option is the most desired, and it is typically reserved for very novel and significant developments. Overall, the goal of this stage is to obtain feedback for your study and incorporate it into your future full manuscript.

Once you have your full data and all the small modifications that are necessary to complete your manuscript, the final stage is the peer-reviewed manuscript. (This is what all projects should strive to complete.) A peer-reviewed manuscript means that your article was reviewed by different individuals in the field, and they delivered comments on the manuscript. The comments were addressed during revision, and then the manuscript was successfully published in a journal in the field, which is indexed into the PubMed database.

The PubMed database is a national database with over 37 million citations of literature and is maintained by the National Center for Biotechnology Information (NCBI) and the United States National Library of Medicine (NLM).[4] It is considered the gold standard of success for a research article. If you get your article accepted to a PubMed-indexed journal, you can be assured that your article will be permanently indexed and available for researchers in the future for use in the medical community.

> Most researchers and investigators only consider PubMed-indexed journals to be "true" publications in the field. Be sure when you are selecting journals that your journal you are submitting too is indexed in PubMed or MEDLINE.

Overall Flow of Ideas: One Last Thought

When considering new ideas, one reading is particularly useful. In 2022, Jeremy Utley and Perry Klebahn, two professors at the prestigious Stanford d.school, published a book titled *Ideaflow: The Only Business Metric That Matters*.[5] In this book, they describe lessons learned while teaching at the d.school and what makes great business entrepreneurs. They provide ample evidence to suggest that good ideas actually come from the quantity of ideas pursued rather than the pursuit of one high-quality idea. In their book, they describe that when individuals pursue many ideas, the chances of one of these ideas resulting in a high-quality and significant finding are higher than focusing on one idea alone. If you are considering ways to bolster your research methodology and formulating ideas, this book is a great read, which is pertinent to our discussion on successfully formulating ideas.

References

1. ArchonMagnus. The scientific method as an ongoing process. August 7, 2025. Accessed at: https://commons.wikimedia.org/wiki/File:The_Scientific_Method_as_an_Ongoing_Process.svg.
2. The New England Journal of Medicine. About NEJM. 2024. Accessed at: https://www.nejm.org/about-nejm/about-nejm.
3. Scimago Journal & Country Rank. 2024. Accessed at: https://www.scimago-jr.com.
4. National Library of Medicine: National Center for Biotechnology Information. PubMed. 2024. Accessed at: https://pubmed.ncbi.nlm.nih.gov.
5. Utley J, Klebahn P. Ideaflow: The only business metric that matters. *Portfolio*. Brentford, Middlesex, United Kingdom. October 25, 2022.

3 Institutional Review Boards

One of the first steps in pursuing a research idea that you formulated is to consider whether you would need a review by the local institution review board. The Institutional Review Board (IRB) was first established in 1974 when the National Research Act was established to ensure the protection of human rights research.[1] This began the requirement of all studies using human subjects to allow for the review of their protocol before implementation.

The IRB is typically located at your local institution and is freely available to faculty members, students, and staff. Third-party individuals and companies wishing to pursue approval by an IRB often have to pay a hefty amount for an IRB review as a third party.

The IRB itself has certain requirements for its sitting members. Every IRB is different at each institution; however, you can expect the review board to consist of <10 members, but the exact number and types of sitting individuals vary from university to university. Most IRBs involve individuals who are scientists and medical doctors; however, they are also required to have some individuals who are not in science and involve individuals who are not affiliated with the university.[2] When the study protocol is submitted to the IRB, these individuals review the application and make sure the study protects the rights and welfare of the human subjects.

Some topics reviewed by the IRB are as follows: Is the sample size large enough to power the study you are trying to perform? Does the study have a rigorous consenting procedure? Are there safeguards in place for any adverse events, and is there a protocol in place for handling sensitive information?

For a new researcher, being familiar with the IRB is crucial, as not conforming to the IRB process can lead to serious consequences, such as denial of the IRB application, rejection of the manuscript for publication, and referral of the investigator to an institutional professionalism committee.

When should you Submit your Study to an Institutional Review Board for Approval?

Per the United States Department of Health and Human Services,[3] research studies should be submitted to the IRB that:

1. Obtains information or biospecimens through intervention or interaction with living individuals and uses, studies, or analyzes the information or biospecimens.

or

2. Obtains, uses, studies, analyzes, or generates identifiable private information or identifiable biospecimens.

Practically speaking, any study that uses human subjects greater than a case report should be submitted for IRB approval. This would include any case series, retrospective reviews, and prospective studies, which should be submitted for IRB approval or acknowledgment. Any participation in multi-center studies should have IRB approval at each site, even if the headquarters site is not at your location. IRBs also continually review the application at specified time points made by the IRB, where the applicant must submit an update on recruitment, adverse events, early termination, or significant findings.

Institutional Review Board Application

In most university settings, an applicant must complete online or in-person basic human subject research training before submitting a proposal. Any of these certificates of required training are sometimes required to be submitted before the submission of an application to an IRB.

When you submit an IRB application, there are three main types of approval you can request:

- **IRB exemption:** Research with very minimal risk to human subjects can be considered exempt from continuing review board approval.
  - Surveys
  - Some quality improvement studies
  - Wellness studies
- **Expedited IRB review:** Research involving no more than minimal risk to subjects, including blood sampling in minimal amounts, review or records collected for non-research purposes, and survey research.
  - Most institutional retrospective reviews of data will fall into this category
- **Convened IRB:** Any study involving greater than minimal risk, including studies with vulnerable populations and/or sensitive questions as well as studies with a possibility of physical risk.
  - Most prospective trials will fall into this category

Even when you question the need for IRB approval, it is always better to submit to an IRB and have the board state the study is exempt. This is better than the reverse scenario, such as being almost complete with a study and not having the appropriate IRB approval. Most journals will require you to have an IRB statement and number in the methods section of the manuscript when submitting for publication. It is important to consider that most national de-identified bases do not need IRB approval, as the information is completely anonymized and publicly available, and there is no way to identify patients in the data.

Completing the Application

When completing the IRB application, the board will request several pieces of data from the team. First, the team will have to declare a principal investigator. This person is responsible entirely for oversight of the study and will answer to any adverse actions obtained by the study. Additionally, the team will need to submit a study protocol or plan. Every member of the study will need to be added to the protocol if that individual is handling patient data. Once submitted, additional people can also be added. However, this typically requires the application to go back to the board for another review of the project.

Retrospective Studies

For retrospective studies, many institutions are able to retro-actively collect patient data in the electronic health record system. This is known as a "chart review," "data collecting," or "data mining." Before performing this process, IRB approval must be secured, but it typically can be secured using an expedited status as it involves minimal risk to patients. The patients have already been treated, therefore any action you do retroactively will be of minimal risk, which is typically considered a risk of a data breach. For these applications, the IRB requires a full set of inclusion and exclusion criteria for the study, including early termination criteria, and they will want you to submit a data collection form with your submission. Another additional hurdle is that in retrospective reviews, patients have typically not consented to the study beforehand. Therefore, in this application, you would need to explain that consent was not obtained and would be difficult to obtain due to no further patient follow-up.

Prospective Studies

For prospective studies, the IRB application is much more encompassing for what is considered a fully convened IRB review. The IRB will request you to produce the full patient consent document that will be provided to the patient for a signature in addition to any other recruiting documents you plan to provide. The IRB typically requests a full set of inclusion and exclusion criteria for the study, including early termination criteria. Early termination criteria would be in place for a prospective study if, after a short point, you realize the treatment you are attempting to test is leading to significantly worse outcomes than the control group. Additional criteria for early termination are if any severe adverse reactions occur to the tested treatment, or if the patient no longer wishes to participate. The IRB will want to see a statistical power analysis performed to make sure you have enough people to measure your anticipated findings but not too many people that you may be unnecessarily or erroneously selecting. If randomized, they will also want information on your investigator and patient blinding protocol. Finally, IRBs will want you to submit a data collection form with your submission.

ClinicalTrials.gov

If your study is a clinical trial, the IRB will also ask you to register your trial on ClinicalTrials.gov (See the registration link in References).[4] ClinicalTrials.gov is a publicly available database where the public can view all clinical trials being performed in the United States. This repository has information on study protocols, results, and any adverse events that may have occurred. Additionally, here, you can find if studies are in the recruiting phases, testing phases, or completed. It is highly encouraged (and sometimes required) to register your clinical trial in this database, as this also helps in preventing duplication of clinical trials. Researchers can use this publicly available data to see if another researcher from another location is performing the same study and to help with not duplicating the trial. ClinicalTrials.gov also aids in disseminating preliminary results of studies as well.

To know if your study is a clinical trial, most institutions use the definition according to the revised common rule 1230.102(b):

> Clinical trial means a research study in which one or more human subjects are prospectively assigned to one or more interventions (which may include placebo or other control) to evaluate the effects of the interventions on biomedical or behavioral health-related outcomes.

Institution-specific Information

Additionally, after this information, some institutions have required specific information that is specific to that institution.

For example, some institutions have a mandatory requirement of a certain percentage of women and minority patients in their treatment groups. If including hospital employees in your study, institutions may often require permission from the head of internal affairs to be submitted with the IRB.

After Submitting the Application

After submission, the time to hear back from the report is different case-by-case. At some institutions, there is a long-running IRB where they meet almost every day. At most institutions, the board will meet monthly or biweekly; therefore, your application should be reviewed at the next open meeting. Additionally, if you opt for an exempt or expedited review, this is sometimes done by one board member and will occur more quickly. For a fully convened IRB, it will take place with all sitting members.

Once the IRB has completed a first review, the reviewers will typically recommend certain revisions to the study protocols. Once submitted and your IRB is accepted, you will place this information along with the IRB number in the methods section of your manuscript. Congratulations!

During and Completion of the Study

Once your IRB is approved, the IRB committee will require an update to the study every 1–2 years. The timeframe is made at the initial review of the application. During these updates, the investigator should update the IRB on any procedure that has been performed, recruitment status, and any results or adverse events that have occurred. Additionally, if an adverse action occurs, this should be submitted to the IRB immediately. Once the study is complete, a finalized closure report is additionally sent to the IRB.

Institutional Animal Care and Use Committee and Institutional Biosafety Committee

You may additionally hear about the Institutional Animal Care and Use Committee in your research-related endeavors. A full explanation of this committee is beyond the scope of this book, but it is essentially the IRB for animal/vertebrate studies. You may also hear of the Institutional Biosafety Committee — this is an IRB similar entity for infectious agents, human and/or non-human primate agents, all modified organisms/plants, and recombinant/synthetic nucleic acids.[5] If you are performing a study that works with any of these specifications, you will have to complete a process similar to an IRB for these entities.

References

1. ExtraNet: Fred Hutch Cancer Center. Institutional Review Board overview. September 10, 2024. Accessed at: https://extranet.fredhutch.org/en/u/irb/institutional-review-board-overview.html#:~:text=On%20July%2012%2C%201974%2C%20the,behavioral%20research%20involving%20human%20subjects.

2. Oregon State University. What is the Institutional Review Board (IRB)? 2024. Accessed at: https://research.oregonstate.edu/irb/what-institutional-review-board-irb#:~:text=The%20Board%20will%20also%20include,periodically%20involved%20in%20protocol%20review.

3. U.S. Department of Health and Human Services: Enhancing the health and well-being of all Americans. Chart 1: Is an activity reseach involving

human subjects? February 16, 2016. Accessed at: https://www.hhs.gov/ohrp/regulations-and-policy/decision-charts-pre-2018/index.html#c1.

4. National Library of Medicine. How to register your study. July 2, 2024. Accessed at: https://clinicaltrials.gov/submit-studies/prs-help/how-register-study.

5. Virginia Tech: Invent the future. Research compliance involving animals, biohazardous agents and/or human subjects. Accessed at: https://www.research.vt.edu/content/dam/research_vt_edu/orc/files/iacuc-irb-ibc-printable.pdf.

Part II
Types of Manuscripts

4 Case Reports and Case Series

Now that you have learned if your study needs IRB approval and, if so, has obtained IRB through the previous steps, how do you know what type of study you will be writing up? In the next four chapters, we will discuss, at an introductory level, the different types of manuscripts you may be exposed to early in your career.

Case Reports

The first and most simple manuscript would be considered a case report. A case report is produced when an author believes they have found a novel presentation of a disease, a novel treatment of a disease, or a novel complication of a disease that has not been previously described in the literature.

Typical presentations of this type of report are when a medical student is on a rotation where an attending physician will perform a novel treatment or have a novel presentation of the disease. Many attendings will suggest to write-up a case report on rounds. This can be a good way to establish a dialog and build a professional relationship with the attending. High-impact case reports can often be in the form of a novel complication of a certain disease, where a new type of treatment for the complication was delivered. If the treatment worked well and without complication, this situation would be a good candidate for a case report.

Case reports can be one of the simplest studies to produce mechanically; however, an extensive search of the PubMed database should be performed before proceeding to manuscript production. This can be performed by typing:

"disease name" and "patient population" and "treatment"

or something similar in PubMed for a more specific search. Be very sure that there is no previously published report on your particular concept of interest. Case reports are simple to perform, but true novel case reports are actually difficult to find. Case reports as an entirety are built on novelty. Therefore, if your case is not novel, most journals will likely reject your case report, and it will fall to lower-tier journals. Additionally, some higher impact factor journals do not accept case reports at all. This is important to discover before submitting your work.

Additionally, it is also worth noting that case reports are not required to have IRB approval. However, most journals will require a completed consent document from the patient to be presented in the report. Always obtain written consent for case reports, as you will most likely need to submit this document along with the report to journals.

> Be sure to search PubMed whether or not your case report is truly novel. If you completely write up a case report, but there is already one previously described on PubMed, it will be INCRED-IBLY difficult to get this published. Oftentimes, in this scenario, case reports are not able to be published at all, and all the time put into developing this manuscript could have been used elsewhere.

Writing a Case Report

The formatting for a case report can deviate somewhat from traditional studies. Case reports will have a much lower maximum number of references (≤20 references as an example) and will often have a much smaller maximum number of words (≤2500 words permitted as an example). They will also have unformally structured abstracts as well.

Case reports will have an introduction that introduces the novel idea being presented. It will also follow with a "History and Physical," much like an actual patient note. Here, the author will explain the clinical history and physical examination findings. It will additionally describe any treatments or surgeries performed on the patients with any pertinent medical dosages, surgical approaches, and any post-operative or treatment complications.

Be sure to include any pertinent and de-identified radiographic, CT, or MRI images pertinent to the case that will be useful for readers. Some case reports, especially in surgical sub-specialties, will include a short operative video to go along with the report. If possible, this is a significant way to boost the acceptability of a case report to a good journal. Additionally, some journals specifically request video submissions. If you are a medical student rotating in a surgical specialty and someone suggests you write a case report, ask if there is any capability of having a video of the surgical approach made, with the patient's consent, of course. With videos, these should be captured in high definition using the MP4 format. With videos, most will need to have an individual narrate the video with computer video-narrating software. There is much software online offering this availability, but it can also be performed for free using iMovie, Windows Movie Maker, or other similar programs.

At the end of the report, it should give the length of the longest follow-up and the overall outcome of the treatment. Lastly, the manuscript will end with a discussion relating your new idea to the current literature, e.g., how does this new finding relate to current studies? How does this case demonstrate that this is an effective treatment technique not described in the literature before? What should treating physicians take home after reading your report? If the case report allows for a conclusion, let the reader know, in one brief paragraph, the overall take-home point of your manuscript. True case reports are very hard to find, but when something truly novel does occur, case reports can introduce new treatment ideas for someone to study in the future.

Case Series

Similar to case reports, case series describe patients with a novel disease presentation, treatment outcome, or adverse event. However, in a case series, there are multiple patients being described. This typically occurs in patients that have somewhat rare disease pathologies where there are multiple patients with the disease but not enough to complete a full retrospective review and perform a comprehensive statistical analysis. These patients are common in very subspecialized surgical fields, as many surgery subspecialties have rare disease pathologies. Essentially, investigators have a need to describe novel cases, but they do not have the total number of patients that would be required to perform a complete retrospective review.

Retrospective cohort studies will oftentimes have a control group (someone who did not undergo the treatment) and will have standardized lengths of follow-up. Case series do not present control groups and may not have standardized lengths of follow-up.

It is important to note that case series generally **do** need IRB approval before capturing patient data and completing a manuscript. This is because there is more than one patient, and it is indeed research on human subjects. Therefore, IRB approval should be approved before handling any patient data when performing a case series.

A strong limitation of case series is that the total n value of the sample size is small (n <20), and even with a small sample size the data quality is generally not as good. Follow-up times are commonly vastly different (if follow-up data is captured at all), and the treatments for each patient are also different, leading to heterogeneous data (data that is not standardized). Institutions can be different, and treating physicians can also be different among patients in case series, which severely limits the quality of data, derived from these reports.

Another significant limitation is the inability to perform statistical tests with these small cohorts. Small samples are not great with statistics, as the power of the sample is not high enough to find differences that occur <5% of the time by chance. Therefore, if you perform statistics on sample sizes with <20 patients, chances are that you will not find any test that is statistically significant. Therefore, case series are often very limited in what they can do; however, if you are studying a patient population with a very small sample size, it may be the best you can do given your data. Case series are typically considered anecdotal evidence and not rigorously standardized or tested.

5 Retrospective Studies

The next higher echelon of conducted studies is retrospective reviews. These are considered more high quality than case reports and case series but of less high quality than prospective studies (Fig. 5.1). Retrospective cohort reviews comprise a large proportion of current medical literature.

The idea for retrospective reviews is simple: In a standardized fashion, an investigator creates strict guidelines for inclusion and exclusion. Typically, this consists of all treatments being standardized, treating providers being standardized, and the treatment setting being standardized to the greatest possible extent. Sometimes, complete standardization of these measures is not possible (for example, when performing a retrospective review of the same procedure being performed by multiple different surgeons). To have the most rigorously standardized studies, one needs to create a prospective study controlling for all of these aforementioned factors.

Nevertheless, much of the medical literature comprises this type of retrospective evidence by gathering data from institutional datasets, national databases, and global databases for certain disease pathologies.

Here, in this chapter, we will discuss how to initially operationalize a retrospective study by picking a data source, obtaining IRB approval, retrieving data, and performing statistical analyses.

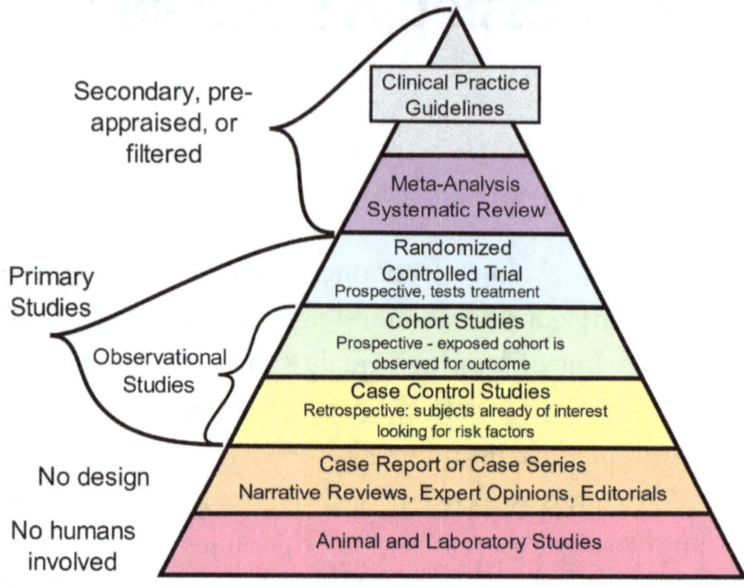

Fig. 5.1.   Hierarchy of evidence-based research.[1]

Picking a Data Source

There are several different types of data sources to choose from. Ultimately, depending on your situation, many of the available options will be limited depending on your institutional affiliation. If you have a smaller institution, the availability of institutional data may be scarce or not be available for usage at all. Sometimes, an institution may have such a long process to approve the use of institutional data that it may not be worth the time and effort to complete this process. Medical students from these institutions are more limited and should seek opportunities using publicly available datasets or collaborate with researchers at institutions with more easily accessible institutional datasets. Individuals from bigger institutions are at an advantage, as they can use pretty much any kind of data source, from having easy access to institutional datasets or even national databases.

Ways to obtain access to institutional data are also often different at each institution, as some institutions employ virtual private networks that are encrypted and rated for IRB usage of privately identifiable information. On this system, students can access the stored data via a virtual private network window on their own computers. Students also can have access to a view-only portion of the electronic health record to retrieve information and store it in the database. Other institutions may have an office that is strictly dedicated to retrieving patient data for retrospective studies once IRB approval is achieved. Whatever types of data you have access to, there should be options to pursue, no matter which institution you are located in. Here, we will discuss potential options for data sources for retrospective reviews, with more detailed information in the later chapters that are specific to each resource.

National Available Cancer Databases

With respect to performing retrospective survival analyses with cancer research, there are two main databases to choose from. The benefit of these databases is that they gather data from patients over a long amount of time (up to 15–20 years after diagnosis). This is often not performed in institutional datasets, which is a significant advantage of national databases. Other advantages are that they are typically free to use for investigators, publicly available, and do not need IRB approval. These can be used by individuals at smaller institutions as well.

National Cancer Database

The American College of Surgeons maintains a database of patients treated for cancer in the National Cancer Database.[2] To be eligible for this database, you must be affiliated with a Commission on Cancer accredited program and must complete an application that includes a letter of support, an online application, and a short proposal of your study. Personal Biosketches are also requested for members of your team as well as a preliminary statistical plan. Once approved, they will send you a large spreadsheet of patients for your particular tumor type. This spreadsheet is known as a Participant-User-File. Using this database does not require IRB approval, as it is systematically de-identified. This resource additionally comes at no cost to the investigator.

This database is an excellent resource for any investigator pursuing studies related to cancer research. As you can easily identify patients with specific types of tumors, you can narrow your search to only those individuals. It gives you case-by-case information where you can perform an adjusted survival analysis, which looks at overall survival and the most recent updates to allow for assessing disease-specific survival. One disadvantage is there is no information on progression-free survival in the National Cancer Database. However, it does include many patient variables, such as age, race, ethnicity, sex, household income, insurance status, marriage status, urban/rural location, use of radiotherapy, use of chemotherapy, time to treatment, and many other disease-specific outcomes. All of the outcomes can be viewed in the National Cancer Database data dictionary.[2] This database is similar to the Surveillance, Epidemiology, and End Results database (see the next section) but is much bigger in size.

Once the process is complete, this is almost a gold standard resource for cancer studies.

Surveillance, Epidemiology, and End Results Database

The National Cancer Institute also publishes a similar database to the National Cancer Database entitled the Surveillance, Epidemiology, and End Results database, otherwise known as SEER.[3] This database is largely similar to the National Cancer Database, except it is smaller in size and has a slightly smaller amount of available variables. The advantage of SEER is that it is very user-friendly, consisting of downloading a program that is used as a portal to retrieve data. Therefore, you can look up any tumor and perform any study without additional application processes. Additionally, this resource does not require IRB approval due to its de-identified nature. This resource also comes at no cost to the investigator.

The application process to initially obtain the SEER*Stats program is simple. You submit an online application but need an endorsement from an official from your school. Subsequently, you download the SEER*Stats program, which is essentially the database portal. One caveat of this program is that it can only be used on a Windows operating system. There are additional databases you can also request access to, including the SEER Medicare database and incidence data with a census tract attributes database. The application for SEER can be found here.[3]

Once downloaded, you will have access to all different types of tumors. It has case-by-case data for investigators to assess overall survival only. There is no information for disease-specific survival or progression-free survival in SEER. A complete detailed annotation of the variables found in SEER can be found via Ref. 4.

National Surgical Quality Improvement Program

The National Surgical Quality Improvement Program is sponsored and produced by the American College of Surgeons and is designed to be a nationally validated, risk-adjusted, outcome-based program designed to improve the quality of surgical care.[5] This database tracks all complications of surgery during the hospital stay and up to 30 days after the surgery. Initially, this program was foreseen to cut down on readmission rates but contained valuable data.

Institutional Datasets

When performing retrospective reviews, institutional datasets are also very useful if available. Typically, institutional datasets are better for measuring more granular and short-term outcomes. For example, in surgery, outcomes like post-operative cranial nerve deficits, 30-day readmission, extended length of stay, and non-routine discharges can all be measured and assessed. These are factors that are too granular to make it into the large national datasets. With institutional datasets, you can also always have the option to go back and add missing variables via an electronic health record search to complete your study. One disadvantage of these datasets, however, is that long-term survival outcomes for cancer are typically not gathered in these datasets. Unless it is a tumor with a low length of survival, many patients will not follow up at the institution after a long period of time.

But how do you get started with institutional datasets? This is largely determined by which institution you are located at. Places with a large amount of resources will typically have a virtual private network system that is secured for storing identifiable information. This can be easily accessed through a researcher's computer. If this is the case, a safe folder should also be created in this system. Use a view-only edition of the electronic health record to retrieve patient data and place the data securely in an Excel file in this safe folder. Many institutions additionally have programs that will search prior records for all patients given a certain diagnosis and any additional criteria you may want to screen for. Imaging additionally can also be retrieved through similar methods in DICOM format.

Before accessing any of this patient-identifiable data, however, the IRB must approve the study. Additionally, many principal investigators have run IRBs to retrieve specific data on an ongoing basis. If you do not have this in your group, having a running IRB for your retrospective data can significantly increase your workflow, as you do not have to spend time submitting IRBs. If you have undergraduate students or junior medical students looking to get involved in medical research, enlist their help in retrieving data while more experienced people perform the statistics and format the manuscripts. It is important to remember that at many of these institutions, the data should not leave the virtual private network environment; therefore, all statistics and analysis should take place through the safe virtual private network as well.

In less robust institutions, a data retrieval office (or an individual person) exists to pull data. This is good for the fact that you can retrieve institutional data, but it is also somewhat limited in that once you submit your query to the office, you are on their timeline for when they respond to your query. This is opposed to if you had direct access yourself, then the timeline is almost completely up to your team. Nevertheless, these data retrieval options are a valuable resource.

Finally, if you go to an institution without any resources to obtain individualized data, there are still options. First, make use of all of the publicly available resources from this book. These can be public databases (there are many), systematic reviews, meta-analyses, and case reports. There are still ample ways to meaningfully contribute using these study formats. Even in places with ample institutional resources, researchers still complete these types of projects because they are still valuable. If you would like to use institutional data, try to collaborate with bigger institutions to assist with their projects or suggest ideas to study.

Additional Data Sources

These aforementioned data sources are some of the most commonly used sources for medical data that you will use in research studies. However, we also provide a complete and comprehensive overview in Chapters 8 to 16 of this book's data sources.

Picking a Statistical Analysis Method

Unlike case series, retrospective reviews have the benefit of being able to perform statistics to measure results. Picking the right (and correct) statistical method is imperative. When performing statistical analysis, there are two broad categories to initially consider. Univariable statistics describe the association of one independent variable with one dependent variable. This is the most basic type of statistical testing. In a multivariable model, the tests take into account multiple independent covariates when describing an association with a dependent variable. This can be known as "adjusting" for additional factors. For example, it could be hypothesized that a high daily intake of sugar could lead to an increased likelihood of obtaining a diagnosis of diabetes. This could be discovered on a bivariable model. However, if we add obesity as an additional factor in the multivariable model, we realize that obesity actually causes diabetes and that it is just more likely that people with high amounts of sugar are also obese, thus making the diabetes diagnosis more likely. We would call this assessing the relationship of sugar with diabetes while adjusting for obesity in our model. It is paramount to learn the difference between bivariable and multivariable modeling. In this section, a brief discussion will be made with which statistical tests are used to answer a specific question. In later chapters, we will specifically introduce how to perform these tests in RStudio with sample coding phrases.

Comparing Baseline Demographics

Initially, we will compare two cohorts in a retrospective study — one cohort with the intervention in question and another cohort without the intervention in question. This cohort would be known as the control group. Initially, we would want to compare baseline differences between the cohorts to make sure they are similar to one another. First, we would need to see if our data is normally distributed or not. This test would be known as the Shapiro–Wilk test for data normality. In normally distributed data, the median = mode, which = mean. An example of normally distributed data would be a tumor that is most common at a certain age and is not as common the further you get from that age. Normally, distributed data is also termed parametric (Fig. 5.2).

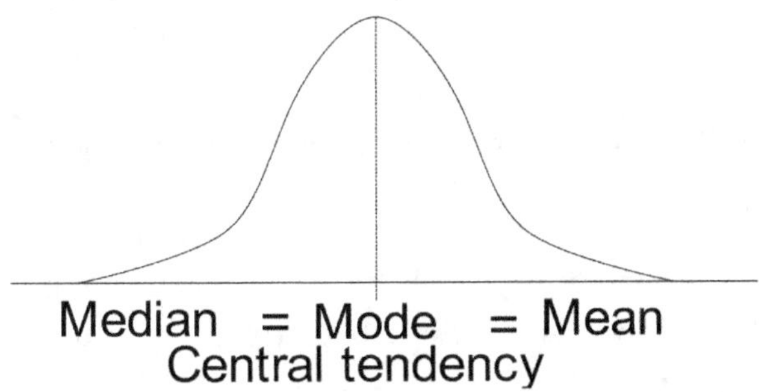

Fig. 5.2.　Example of a normally distributed dataset.[6]

Non-parametric data, on the other hand, is when all of the above are not true. Consider a survival curve like the following figure. Here, you can see the mean > median > mode, and by a large amount. This would be considered non-parametric data (Fig. 5.3).

This is important because the statistical tests you use for comparing averages will be different, given whichever type of data you have. Mean values in your baseline cohorts should be compared

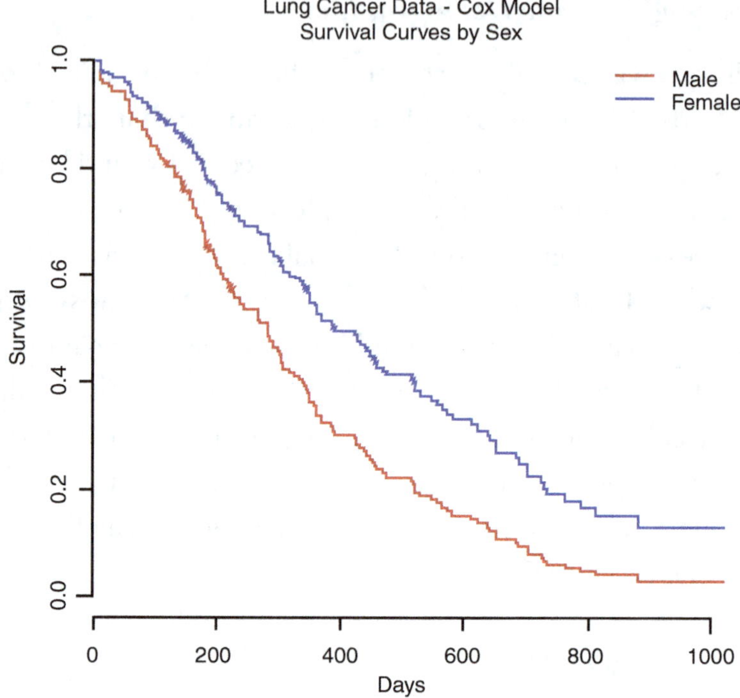

Fig. 5.3.   Example of a non-normally distributed dataset.[7]

with the student's t-test for parametric data, and it should be compared with the Mann–Whitney U test for non-parametric data.

For categorical data, comparisons will be made with the chi-squared test, generally for n-values with n >30, and Fischer's exact test for n-values <30.

As you can see in the following table, we are comparing the baseline demographics for two cohorts — one cohort that underwent surgery and the other cohort that did not undergo surgery. The mean age was compared with the student's t-tests, and it was found to be different in statistical significance. Months from diagnosis to treatment were compared using the Mann–Whitney U test, as it was found not normally distributed. Sex, race, ethnicity, household income, residence, chemotherapy, and radiotherapy were placed as categorical variables and compared with chi-squared testing since n >30 for each variable. Only radiotherapy was found to be statistically different between the two baseline cohorts. All of these tests would be considered bivariable testing since we are not adjusting for additional covariates in our model. When performing a retrospective study, it is imperative to compare baseline demographics from each of your cohorts (Table 5.1).

Table 5.1. Baseline Cohort Comparisons of Patients Receiving Surgical Recommendation for a Tumor

Characteristics	Surgery (N = 2198)	Did not undergo surgery (N = 163)	P
Mean age (years)	34 ± 14	40 ± 16	<0.001
Sex			0.801
Female	888 (40.4)	68 (41.7)	
Male	1310 (59.6)	95 (58.3)	
Race			0.736
White	1819 (82.8)	144 (88.3)	
Black	238 (10.8)	13 (8.0)	
Asian or Pacific Islander	105 (4.8)	4 (2.5)	
American Indian/Alaska Native	6 (0.3)	2 (1.2)	
Ethnicity			0.690
Hispanic	386 (17.5)	20 (12.3)	
Not hispanic	1714 (80.0)	138 (84.6)	
Unknown	98 (4.5)	5 (3.1)	
Median household income			
<$50 k/year			0.678
≥$50 k/year	1180 (53.7)	73 (44.8)	
Unknown	813 (37.0)	67 (41.1)	
	205 (9.3)	23 (14.1)	

(Continued)

Table 5.1.   (*Continued*)

Characteristics	Surgery (N = 2198)	Did not undergo surgery (N = 163)	P
Residence			0.194
Rural	42 (2.0)	3 (1.8)	
Urban	2052 (93.3)	147 (90.2)	
Unknown	104 (4.7)	13 (8.0)	
Months from diagnosis to initial treatment[2]	0 ± 1	2 ± 2	<0.001
Chemotherapy			0.228
Received	825 (37.5)	91 (55.8)	
Did not receive	1349 (61.4)	71 (43.6)	
Unknown	24 (1.1)	1 (0.6)	
Radiation			<0.001
Received	1689 (76.8)	100 (61.3)	
Did not receive	378 (17.2)	56 (34.4)	
Unknown	122 (5.6)	7 (4.3)	

[1]Median [95% CI] Survival Time in Months calculated with the Kaplan–Meier method and compared with a log-rank test.
[2]Initial receipt of surgical resection, chemotherapy, or radiation.

Initial Comparisons

Initial comparisons will typically be performed with a logistic or linear regression. Logistic regression compares the likelihood of one categorical variable being associated with another categorical variable. Linear regression compares a continuous variable with a categorical variable. For example, consider the following table comparing our same variables with whether surgery succeeded in benefiting the patient (Table 5.2). In your study, replace any of your desired outcomes with successful treatment. Linear regression was used to determine whether increasing age was associated with successful treatment. Here, it was not, as it had an odds ratio of 0.97 and was statistically significant. The second brackets are confidence

Table 5.2. Bivariable and Multivariable Comparisons

	Univariable logistic regression		Multivariable logistic regression	
	Odds ratio [95% CI]	**P**	**Adjusted odds ratio [95% CI]**	**P**
Surgical recommendation				
Age	0.97 [0.96–0.98]	<0.001	0.97 [0.97–0.99]	<0.001
Sex				
Male	Reference		Reference	
Female	0.95 [0.69–1.31]	0.737	0.92 [0.64–1.32]	0.647
Race				
White	Reference		Reference	
Asian/Pacific Islander	1.45 [0.52–6.00]	0.534	/	0.973
Black	1.45 [0.84–2.73]	0.207	1.47 [0.82–2.88]	0.222
Ethnicity				
Not hispanic	Reference		Reference	
Hispanic	1.69 [0.35–30.4]	0.609	0.89 [0.15–16.7]	0.910
Marital status				
Not married				
Married				
Median household income				
<$50 k/year	Reference		Reference	
≥$50 k/year	1.12 [0.81–1.54]	0.501	1.18 [0.83–1.69]	0.361
Total number of tumors				

intervals, which describe a 95%-confidence interval. Therefore, we are certain to have a 95%-level of confidence that our true odds ratio is between 0.96 and 0.98. Therefore, this is a strong confidence interval as it is not very wide. Logistic regression was used to determine if sex was associated with successful treatment, and it was not, as it was not statistically significant. It is also important to note that in tables, the variable with the odds ratio data is always compared to its reference line. The p-value denotes the level of significance. Most clinical studies will incorporate a threshold of p <0.05 as a threshold for determining statistical significance. This means we have a less than 5% chance that our finding was due to randomness.

Adjusted Comparisons

Adjusted comparisons, also called multivariable comparisons, are similar to the aforementioned comparisons. However, they take into account ALL of the variables on the table. As we can see here, the multivariable model does not show any variables that are not statistically significant that were significant without adjusting. Sometimes, adding variables to a regression model will make another one that was not significant previously significant now. This is called a **suppressor** variable. Sometimes, adding a variable will make an already statistically significant variable no longer significant. This is also normal.

You may be curious how these tests are performed. We will discuss performing these tests using a very common type of statistical program, RStudio, in later chapters. We will also provide actual sample codes for you to use in your assessments.

Survival Analysis

Important considerations when performing survival analysis are the three types of outcomes you can assess. From the least to most important are overall survival, disease-specific survival, and progression-free survival. Overall survival is the measure of a patient with cancer who has died for any reason, even if completely unrelated to the cancer itself. Disease-specific survival is the measure of whether a patient died due to only the cancer. Progression-free survival is a measure of tumor recurrence in a patient and does not inherently indicate the patient is deceased. This is also known as recurrence. These are annotated OS, DSS, and PFS, respectively, with DSS and PFS being more difficult to measure and record, inclusive of national databases. When possible, you should attempt to always measure PFS, but you may only have data for OSS or DSS.

Statistical Models

Studies measuring survival outcomes, also known as time-to-event data, are very similar to what is described above. We will discuss differences here. Of note, there are other instances in which we would use time-to-event data, such as measuring time-to-infection after using a new surgical drainage system. In this reading, we will solely discuss time-to-event data, where it has to do with patient survival, but just know it can be applicable in other areas as well.

Instead of having a bivariable logistic or linear regression, the bivariable form for a survival analysis is termed **log-rank tests**. Instead of having a standardized cut-off like in our logistic and linear regression, the log-rank tests incorporate different follow-up times for each data value; thus, the data is censored. Consider doing an analysis where patients have different lengths of follow-up, and consider one treatment arm where almost all patients are still alive at the follow-up, while in another treatment arm, almost all patients are deceased. At first glance, and with logistic regression, you would see that patients in the later treatment arm had poorer survival when compared to the first treatment arm.

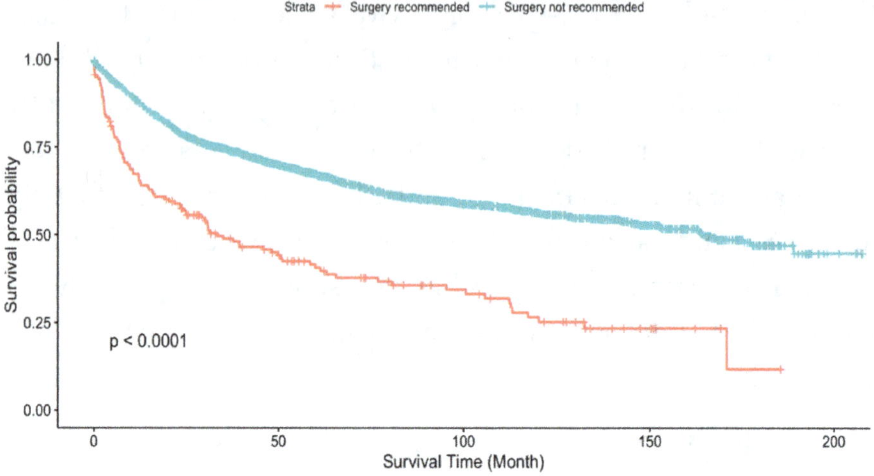

Fig. 5.4.   Bivariable survival assessments using log-rank tests.

However, upon further examination, you realize that most patients in the first treatment arm were evaluated two weeks after treatment, while the patients in the later arm were evaluated five years after treatment. Therefore, the patients in the first group had poorer survival than the later group. Accounting for the differences in follow-up times is what is performed in the log-rank tests (Fig. 5.4). Instead of reporting values in relative risk or odds ratio, the hazard is reported in a hazard ratio (HR).

One final model we will additionally be discussing is the Cox proportional hazards model. This is a common multivariable model for time-to-event data. It is essentially the multivariable model for the log-rank tests. However, the Cox assumption of this model states that hazards are proportional to survival throughout the timeframe being studied. The outcomes are reported as hazard ratios in this multivariable survival model (Table 5.3).

Table 5.3. Multivariable Cox Proportional Hazards Models for Patients under Resection of Tumor

Characteristics	Hazard ratio	5% lower bound confidence interval	95% upper bound confidence interval	P
Race				
White	Reference	—	—	—
Black	1.057	0.521	4.292	0.938
Asian or Pacific Islander	0.909	0.260	1.586	0.737
Median household income				
<$35,000/year				
$35,000–$44,999	Reference	—	—	—
$45,000–$64,999	1.327	0.137	12.823	0.807
≥$75,000/year	0.404	0.054	3.021	0.377
	0.304	0.041	2.233	0.242
Marital status				
Married	Reference	—	—	—
Not married	1.304	0.922	1.843	0.133
Residence				
Urban	Reference	—	—	—
Rural	1.444	0.812	2.570	0.211

Important Considerations for Statistical Models

When performing statistical models, it is best to consider some main points. First, you can measure the accuracies of statistical models using a c-statistic or an area under the curve assessment. This can be performed in RStudio and will be discussed further in later chapters. Additionally, it is also important to consider variance influence factors and to make sure they are <5. Having high variance influence factors could be an indication of multicollinearity in your model, which means that some variables are almost exactly correlated with one another.

Finally, when performing a multivariable analysis, it is important not to have an overfit statistical model. An overfit model is when there are too many variables introduced into the model, but yet the model has too few patients. The result is the statistical model is trained to the specific randomness of your dataset and will overall lower the accuracy and generalizability of your findings. To combat this issue, we follow the rule of tens for multivariable models. This rule states that for every variable introduced into the multivariable model, we need ten events in the patients. For example, if we want to make a multivariable survival model incorporating age, obesity, sex, hypertension, and smoking, these are five variables, and we would need a dataset of at least 50 patients who are deceased.

Making a Great Retrospective Study

It is important to know that the most useful part of a retrospective study is to have similar baseline demographics between your two comparative cohorts and additionally show changes in your treatment group using an adjusted model. Showing the difference in an unadjusted model may be somewhat novel, but if you can show that it is statistically significant in an adjusted model, this is a very good finding and will generally get your paper accepted to a decent journal.

Discussion and Conclusions

Congratulations! You are now finished with your retrospective review. These are traditional studies that can suggest associations between a specific treatment and a disease outcome. Limitations of these studies are that they are not able to prove the causation of a variable with an outcome as they are not retrospective in etiology, and not all other variables are completely controlled from cohort to cohort. In the discussion, be sure to correlate each of your statistically significant findings with the current literature. In your conclusion, be sure to state what you believe your newly found association may be.

References

1. Pamputt. Research design and evidence. August 3, 2021. Accessed at: https://commons.wikimedia.org/wiki/File:Research_design_and_evidence.svg.

2. American College of Surgeons. Participant user files. 2024. Accessed at: https://www.facs.org/quality-programs/cancer-programs/national-cancer-database/puf/.

3. National Cancer Institute. How to request access to SEER data. Accessed at: https://seer.cancer.gov/data/access.html.

4. National Cancer Institute. Dictionary of SEER*Stat variables. November, 2020. Accessed at: https://seer.cancer.gov/data-software/documentation/seerstat/nov2020/seerstat-variable-dictionary-nov2020.pdf.

5. American College of Surgeons. ACS National Surgical Quality Improvement Program. 2024. Accessed at: https://www.facs.org/quality-programs/data-and-registries/acs-nsqip/.

6. Pk0001. Normal-data. September 15, 2019. Accessed at: https://commons.wikimedia.org/wiki/File:Normal-data.svg.

7. Yosi Levy. Lung cancer cox. November 20, 2018. Accessed at: https://commons.wikimedia.org/wiki/File:Lung_cancer_cox.jpg.

6 Prospective Studies

Now that we have covered some case reports, case series, and retrospective reviews, we will address a type of study higher up on the research hierarchy. Instead of retrospectively reviewing data and performing statistical analysis, prospective studies assess outcomes that will occur in the future. Here, investigators design a study protocol usually involving one treatment cohort and one control cohort that will be enrolled in a prospective fashion. Here, patients will be fully consented to the study of its risks and benefits to society before enrolling. When an investigator randomly assigns patients to a control cohort and to a treatment cohort, this is termed a randomized controlled trial. This is the gold standard type of study that can be performed to assess a medical intervention, and it can also be performed using multiple centers. These types of studies often are accepted by high-impact journals.

Prospective studies are useful to an investigator, as you can only really assess associations that have occurred in the past between an intervention and an outcome in retrospective studies. Therefore, causation cannot really be commented on in retrospective studies. For example, you may find an association with Asian patients having higher survival outcomes via a retrospective study; however, if you strictly control for ability and access to care in a prospective study, you may see this association deteriorate. Thus, being Asian may not necessarily cause increased survival outcomes in cancer.

Some additional terms you may encounter are randomized studies. This occurs when you accrue patients into your prospective study and randomly place patients in the treatment cohort or the control cohort. This attempts to reduce bias by the investigators. Additional terminology includes patient-blind studies and investigator-blind studies. The first refers to whether the patient does not know whether they received the intervention or not (for example, an injection with only saline versus an intervention product), and an investigator blind refers to the investigator not knowing who has the real treatment versus a sham treatment. When both occur in a study, it is noted to be a double-blind study.

When performing prospective studies, the gold-standard product would typically be a randomized controlled trial, which incorporates randomization, a control group, and also patient and investigator blinding. It is important to note that not every study can have all of these features. For example, it would be difficult to patient blind in a study that is assessing a new intervention for brain tumor surgical resection. However, most investigators will attempt to have this feature where possible.

Multi-Center Studies

Often, when performing prospective studies, multiple sites can be used in the study. Therefore, investigators from each institution assess the same intervention prospectively and then submit the data to a central principal investigator. This has several advantages. First, some diseases may have a small sample size with one institution only; therefore, this helps create a larger sample size to assess the intervention.

Second, this helps with study generalizability. Not every type of treatment is the same across different institutions, states, and countries; therefore, if you include institutions from different locations, this makes your study's results more generalizable to a wider population.

Institutional Review Board

All prospective studies will need to be submitted to the Institutional Review Board (IRB). You will generally need a central IRB submission at the main study site in addition to an IRB submission at each other's secondary site as well. In some cases, a data-use agreement can be made where a single-site IRB can monitor the entire trial at other sites. However, this is often on an institution-by-institution basis.

Obtaining Funding

Finally, prospective studies can be difficult to perform, as they typically will require funding. Funding may not be required for the previously aforementioned study types, such as retrospective reviews; however, prospective studies often require salaries paid for research coordinators who schedule patient appointments and collect data in a prospective fashion. Additionally, some prospective studies may also provide compensation to participants as well. Salaries and wages are also required for other personnel who are responsible for consenting the patient, administering data collection, and being responsible for securely storing data. Prospective studies can be difficult to perform, but once performed, could lead to high-impact publications.

7 Performing Systematic Reviews and Meta-Analyses

Sometimes, when investigating a treatment option for a disease, it is crucial to search and compile all previous studies of the disease into one single manuscript. When you follow a standardized search criterion and gather data through a standardized process, it is termed a "systematic review" of the literature. When you take all of these studies together and perform a statistical analysis of data across multiple studies, it is called a "meta-analysis."

These studies are crucial in modern scientific literature, as they summarize all previous work on a given topic and result in a conclusion based on all prior literature published to date. These can have very meaningful results, but they are often studies that are long and cumbersome. In this chapter, we will discuss how to perform a systematic review and meta-analysis.

Searching for Studies

Searching for studies using a systematic review should involve a very rigid and standardized screening method. Ideally, this search protocol would be designed to capture every bit of information on a particular topic. Keep in mind that large search criteria can result in a very long and tedious screening process that can significantly prolong your search time. Alternatively, making your search criteria too narrow can result in you not obtaining enough data to make any significant conclusions.

Search Criteria

Let's say you underwent the idea creation process discussed in Chapter 2 and would like to compile all evidence for a new treatment of diabetic patients with type 1 diabetes. Let's assume that there have been six retrospective reviews assessing this treatment published in the literature. Systematic reviews and meta-analyses use previously published data; therefore, these studies do not require IRB approval before beginning a systematic review and meta-analysis.

To get started, we need to develop our strict search criteria, which will be listed in the methods section of our manuscript. For this, we will include the terms "drug name" and "diabetes" and input them directly into PubMed. This is an easy-to-use search term in PubMed, which will pull all studies that include both of these terms in our search results. Additional options could be ("drug name" or "diabetes"); however, this would extend our search results, which may be more difficult for us to screen later on in the process (Fig. 7.1).

When performing our systematic review, we need to adhere to the Preferred Reporting Items for Systematic Review and Meta-Analyses[1] (PRISMA) guidelines (see Appendix 1).

Therefore, in our search, we must include all inclusion and exclusion criteria for the studies we are aiming to capture in

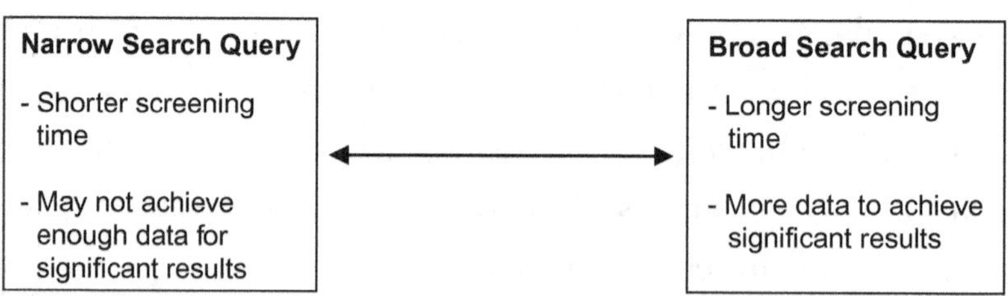

Fig. 7.1.   Spectrum of initial search queries.

our review. Additionally, we will explain and explicitly annotate the search strategy for each of our databases. Common databases will include PubMed, Scopus, Web of Science, Google Scholar, Embase, EBSCO, and Cochrane Library databases. Additionally, the date that the search was performed should be annotated in the Methods section, as well as the date range searched in the same section. Keep in mind that many healthcare treatment options have significantly changed over time; therefore, some authors of systematic reviews limit searches to the most recent 10 years.

Screening

Strict inclusion and exclusion criteria should be annotated in the Methods section. In this section, you can specify whether you are using data from peer-reviewed manuscripts only or also including data presented at conference presentations. Typical things to exclude would be letters (non-peer-reviewed), editorials (non-peer-reviewed), literature reviews with no patient data, and studies that involve the same principal investigator or institution (to avoid patient duplication). In this later scenario, you would only include the larger study. Additionally, conference reports can also be accepted; however, keep in mind this is typically preliminary data, and it also may be duplicate data from other fully published manuscripts. At any point, it is better to err on the side of caution and exclude any study that may be in question.

To screen the articles, it is best to use two individual screeners while having a third author make a decision from articles that have screening results with conflicting opinions. This tie-breaking author would generally be a more senior author. The screening process typically occurs via the title and abstract screen initially and then followed by a full-text screen. Both stages are typically performed with two screeners. Additionally, there are several websites that can be used to assist in this screening process. One prominent website is called Covidence,[2] which has the ability to import articles directly from databases, and it acts to streamline article screening and data extraction capabilities all within one easy-to-use website. This website does have a cost, but several institutions subscribe to this website for their students. Additionally, if you prefer not to take this route, it can also be performed on PubMed manually with simple Excel spreadsheets. The screening process should consider solely inclusion and exclusion criteria determined before beginning the study, and this protocol should be explicitly stated in the Methods section of your manuscript. Once complete, a PRISMA flow diagram should be placed into the manuscript, similar to Fig. 7.2.

In this flow diagram, all databases should be listed at the top of the flow diagram, and the n-values for each particular box should be placed in each box. Generally speaking, all systematic review manuscripts should involve this PRISMA flow diagram, according to PRISMA guidelines.

Data Extraction

When extracting data, the same two-person system should also be employed. Extracted variables should be determined before beginning the study, and all clinical variables should be explicitly described in the Methods section of the manuscript. Additionally, it is important to keep all of the variables consistent throughout each of the studies. For example, if only one study reports blood loss in liters but the majority of studies describe blood loss in milliliters, be sure to convert all variables to a standardized unit.

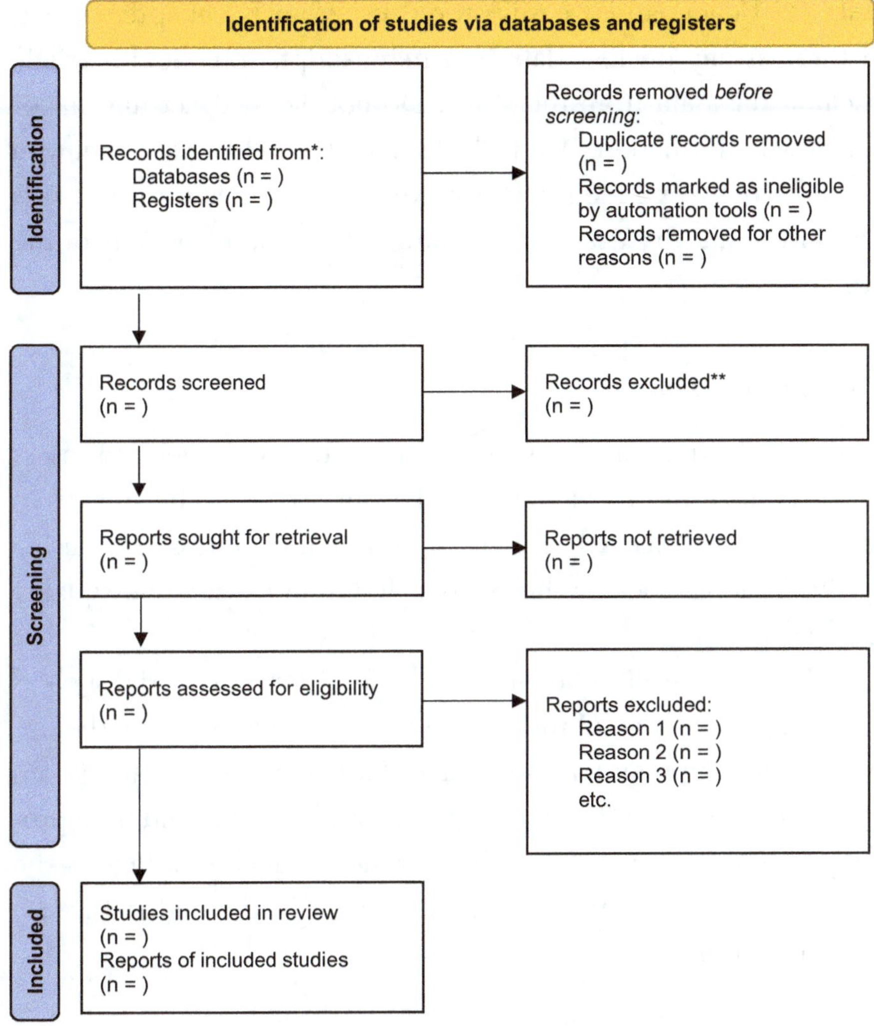

Fig. 7.2. PRISMA flow diagram.

*Consider if feasible to do so, reporting the number of records identified from each database or register searched (rather than the total number across all databases/registers).

**If automation tools were used, indicate how many records were excluded by a human and how many were excluded by automation tools.

Extracted data can be easily stored using an Excel spreadsheet. If there is any unclear data in a manuscript, you should strictly exclude this data from the study. Do not ever extract unclear or unknown information. If a study does not have clear data, then you should strictly exclude the study from the systematic review. It is also important to extract any funding information from any of the studies as well.

Quality Assessment

Additionally, there are two types of bias you would need to assess when completing meta-analyses. The first type is the quality of the included studies. This is most commonly addressed by using quality scoring, such as the Newcastle-Ottawa Guidelines quality grading system.[3]

This rates each individual study on different criteria, such as being representative of the regular population as a whole, the use of control groups, and the adequacy of follow-up. After rating each study, you can consider reporting each study's rating and then providing an average of your included studies' quality ratings in the results section of your publication. Obviously, the higher the rating, the better.

Publication Bias

Once this is performed, the next type of bias that should be addressed is publication bias. Generally speaking, if you think about the world of publishing, you would assume that most investigators publish both results that show statistical differences and additional results that show null results, but, in reality, it can often occur that studies with significant results are published more than

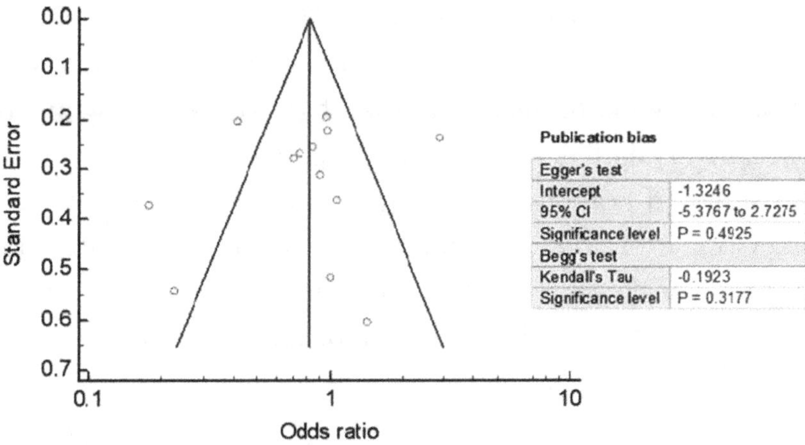

Fig. 7.3.   Funnel plot for publication bias.[4]

studies with null results. This can be due to the lack of investigators submitting null results for publication, and it can also occur if journals are less likely to accept studies without significant findings. When this type of bias occurs, it is termed publication bias. One way to screen for this is by using funnel plots. Consider the funnel plot in Fig. 7.3.

Here, we can see this is a test for odds ratio, with odds ratio values on the x-axis and standard error values on the y-axis. Additionally, there is a funnel shape in the middle of the figure. This funnel shape occurs since studies with smaller standard errors are studies with larger sample sizes; thus, there are fewer leniencies for randomness. At the bottom with the larger standard error values, these are small studies; therefore, there is more leniencies for random results, and the funnel fans outwards. Each yellow circle on the figure is a study that corresponds to the observed odds ratio value in addition to the standard error. Studies that are located outside of the funnel are termed outliers, and the lines on the funnel are 95% confidence intervals.

The way we assess for publication bias is by plotting all studies onto a funnel plot, and once we have plotted all studies, we observe the funnel to make sure that the variables are symmetrically occurring both at the smaller standard error values and at the larger standard error values. In Fig. 7.3, this is the case. You can actually run a p-value for funnel plots that will detect publication bias. In this test, the p-value was not significant, and the studies are symmetric; therefore, this is an indication that no publication bias may be occurring.

However, if your meta-analysis depicted a funnel plot that was asymmetric, with fewer smaller studies being published for specific findings, this could be an indication of publication bias. Alternatively, consider Fig. 7.4. In this funnel plot, we can see evidence of asymmetry. Here, we can see fewer smaller studies are being published that have positive results. When looking at the larger studies, there is evidence that the true ln ES is near –0.01 based on the large study annotated at the top. However, only smaller studies with results near –0.05 were published. Additionally, it appears no smaller study with positive values was

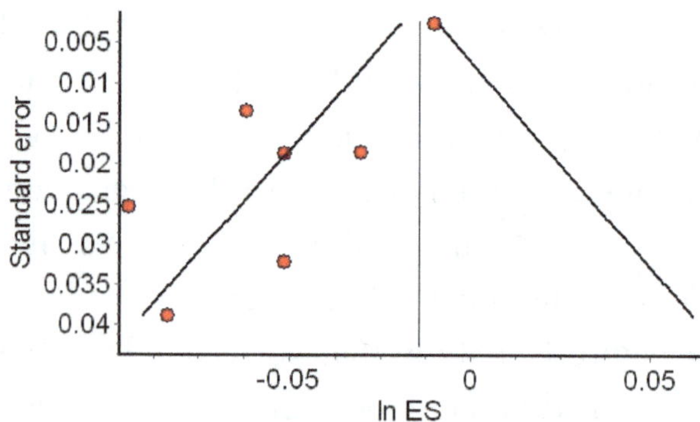

Fig. 7.4.   Example of a funnel plot used in meta-analysis to detect publication bias and depict asymmetry.[5]

published. This would be an indication of possible publication bias and should be annotated in your manuscript.

Both the quality of included studies and publication bias should be annotated in your manuscript. How to actually perform tests for publication bias will be specifically addressed later in Chapter 19.

Reporting Results

When reporting results for your study, you should, at a minimum, have a table with all, including studies, using references. Additionally, you should also include the study's author name, number of patients, nationality of study, basic demographics, and outcomes assessed in the tables, if possible. Once you have all this data tabulated, you must determine whether your systematic review has sufficient and granular data to where a meta-analysis of the data can be performed. If your studies contain too many variables that are not standardized — they include small sample sizes or are too heterogeneous, then a meta-analysis may not be feasible. As a rule of thumb, it is often better to have a strong systematic review compared to a poor meta-analysis. A meta-analysis is performed when you take statistics and apply them to your studies contained in a systematic review.

When assessing direct outcomes, forest plots are used to perform meta-analyses. As you can see in Fig. 7.5, each study is aligned along the y-axis, and the result of each study is aligned along the x-axis. Each black square denotes a study, with the long lines denoting 95% confidence intervals. Specific information is also displayed on the right side of the figure. The shorter the line of the study, the smaller the confidence interval, and the bigger the study.

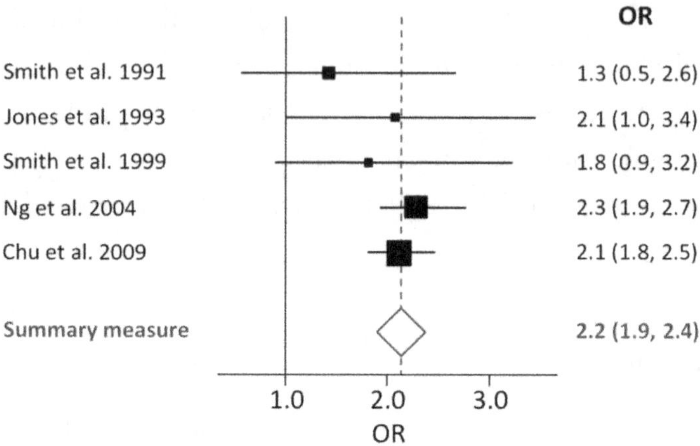

Fig. 7.5. Generic forest plot.[6]

Finally, at the bottom of the figure is the summary measure inclusive of all the above studies. This is termed a meta-analysis.

Random Effects Model Versus Fixed Effects Model

One important concept to understand when meta-analyzing is the concept of heterogeneity. Some comparisons among studies may be very straightforward. Consider studies that measure the effect of lisinopril on a population. This study is likely to be very homogeneous as most patients will likely undergo assessment using the same lisinopril 20 mg medication at every institution, thus resulting in an x amount of decrease in blood pressure that is likely similar among all patients. The pills are the same among all participants, as well as the likelihood of the age of the participants (older). Also, they may likely suffer from metabolic disease or have a genetic predisposition. They are all generally treated with the same pill and will result in a similar reduction of blood pressure across the board. This would be considered homogeneity among studies.

Alternatively, consider performing a meta-analysis of studies using a very specialized and novel surgery such as a craniotomy. When assessing these studies, they are likely to be heterogeneous, as they will be performed in different types of operating rooms with different surgeon techniques, operating room tools, and types of pathologies in question. These heterogeneity assessments can be specifically compared with I^2 values when performing meta-analyses.

When performing a meta-analysis on studies with a homogeneous data distribution ($I^2 <50$), a fixed effects method should be employed. When performing a meta-analysis on studies with a heterogeneous data distribution, a mixed effects model should be employed ($I^2 >50$). Specifics on how to perform these individual studies in RStudio will be discussed in Chapter 20.

Discussion and Conclusions

Congratulations! You are now finished with your first meta-analysis. The significance of these studies is that they use data from multiple different studies to produce an overall conclusion on this type of treatment paradigm. In the discussion, be sure to correlate each of your statistically significant findings with the current literature. In your conclusion, be sure to state what your meta-analysis has found that each individual study by them did not find.

References

1. Page MJ, McKenzie JE, Bossuyt PM, Boutron I, Hoffmann TC, Mulrow CD, *et al.* The PRISMA 2020 statement: An updated guideline for reporting systematic reviews. *British Medical Journal*, 2021; **372**: n71.
2. Covidence. Main webpage. Accessed at: https://www.covidence.org.

3. Newcastle-Ottawa Quality Assessment Scale. Accessed at: https://www.ohri.ca/programs/clinical_epidemiology/nosgen.pdf.

4. Wang J, Xie D, Cai Z, *et al*. Does a home-based exercise program play any role in the treatment of knee osteoarthritis? A meta-analysis. *Adv Clin Exp Med*. 2022; **31**(11): 1187–1196.

5. Sardmetal. Funnel plot depicting asymmetry. September 27, 2015. Accessed at: https://commons.wikimedia.org/wiki/File:Funnel_plot_depicting_asymmetry_Sept_2015.jpg.

6. James Grellier. Generic forest plot. May 4, 2010. Accessed at: https://commons.wikimedia.org/wiki/File:Generic_forest_plot.png.

Part III
Sources of Data

8 Institutional Datasets

One of the most granular types of datasets that you will be able to use is local institutional datasets. With this type of data source, depending on your institutional infrastructure, you can essentially look up any aspect of a patient's chart and include it in your study. These types of data sources are good, as you can include anything that was ever documented on a patient's chart in your research study.

This type of data source is very useful for short-term cause-and-effect studies and is less strong than databases for measuring long-term survival outcomes. This is because not every patient will follow up with your department until disease progression or death.

In this chapter, we will discuss the use of institutional datasets and how to formulate optimal manuscripts with this source.

Obtaining the Data

This process is different for each institution. Generally speaking, before data is acquired, this type of study must be approved by an institutional review board (IRB) due to the identified nature of the records. More on applying for IRBs can be found in Chapter 3; however, it is generally recommended that all retrospective reviews be IRB-approved beforehand.

Once you have IRB approval, data will be acquired by a manual chart review of a patient's record. This will occur with a clinician or a researcher with read-only access to patient data after a search for patients with a particular disease. Once this information is retrieved, this information should be annotated into an Excel document. This document should ideally be stored on a virtual private network server that is encrypted and protected from outside parties. Some institutions have dedicated offices to perform these reviews. Many institutions also have dedicated software to populate patients with certain pathology, such as the Slicer software.[1] Once you perform data extraction and have built your Excel spreadsheet, keep the database and continually update it! You may need IRB approval for a long-standing database, but this would be the most time-efficient use of your time! Just be sure it is stored in a de-identified manner and on a secured server.

Type of Data to Extract

When extracting patient data, you want to be sure to acquire basic demographical variables in all reviews. For example, you should almost always include a patient's sex, age, race, and ethnicity (Hispanic or non-Hispanic) at a minimum. Additional demographic information can include income, education status, geographic location, year of diagnosis, comorbidities, and frailty status using one of the common frailty indices, such as the mFI-5 scale (Table 8.1). Obtaining these items is ideal for each cohort, ideally with both the treatment cohort and control cohort having similar baseline demographics.

Table 8.1. mFI-5 Criteria

Item	Score
History of diabetes mellitus	1 or 0
Congestive heart failure within 30 days	1 or 0
Hypertension requiring medication	1 or 0
History of COPD or pneumonia	1 or 0
Functional status: Partially dependent or totally dependent	1 or 0

Once you obtain all of these variables for each patient, format your Excel spreadsheet to include columns with the item name at the top of each column and each patient as a row. In each cell, you will include a "1" or a "0" in the cell for categorical variables and numerics for continuous variables. Do not leave any cell blank, as this will cause issues later on with the statistics and will often require a re-review of the patients. There is a difference between "0" and a cell left blank in terms of running statistics.

Once you have these basic demographical variables recorded, you can then add columns for the treatment outcomes you are attempting to measure. You can essentially measure anything that is in your hypothesis, and you would simply enter the treatment as a "1" or a "0" for having "occurred" versus "not occurred," respectively. Once the treatment is gathered, you can then enter outcomes. Retrospective studies may measure the following short-term outcomes (Table 8.2).

Lastly, one of the most important outcomes to include is the length of follow-up. Generally speaking, you would want to make it standardized among all patients in your review. Measuring the rate of post-operative infections among patients can be very different if you are measuring some patients a day after being released from the hospital versus 29 days after leaving the hospital. Attempt to make your follow-up length as standardized as possible.

Table 8.2. Typical Short-Term Outcomes in Retrospective Reviews

Item	Description
30-day re-admission	Whether the patient was re-admitted to the hospital within 30 days after treatment.
Non-routine discharge	Whether the patient was discharged to a location that is not home.
High hospital costs	Whether the patient incurred over a specific number of hospital costs being measured in the study.
Length of hospital stay	Length of hospital stay in days.

Limitations of Institutional Datasets

Even though these types of studies can provide very granular and detailed data, they are also susceptible to a number of limitations. First, most of these institutional datasets do not offer complete follow-ups for patients. For example, if you are studying patients with pancreatic tumors being resected by a general surgery department, there is a good chance that the general surgery department has not followed the patient until death and likely does not have that data in the system. Therefore, this type of data is optimal for when short-term and granular data is needed.

Another limitation is that with rare diseases, there are often not enough patients to make any meaningful conclusions based on one institutional set. Hence, this is why many national and multicenter registries have been created. It may be difficult to find enough patients at your own institution to have any statistically significant and meaningful results.

Finally, institutional datasets are often not generalizable across the globe or even across the United States. For example, rates of short-term adverse outcomes are likely to be significantly different if performing an institutional review in the southeastern United States versus performing a review in other locations of the United States. Thus, it is not as generalizable as national or international database studies can be.

Reference

1. UC Davis Health. Epic — SlicerDicer. 2024. Accessed at: https://health.ucdavis.edu/data/epic-slicer-dicer.html.

9 National Cancer Database

For studies involving cancer patients, the National Cancer Database is an excellent resource.[1] Sponsored by the American College of Surgeons and the Commission on Cancer, the National Cancer database collects data from multiple cancer centers in the United States. This data is provided in organ-specific data sheets, otherwise known as Participant User Files (PUFs), and is one of the largest case-by-case datasets for cancer patients in the United States. This database is excellent for producing studies that assess long-term outcomes in cancer patients while assessing multiple independent data variables for association with outcomes. This database captures overall survival (death from any cause) only and not cancer recurrence (progression-free survival) or death from that particular disease (disease-specific survival).

Obtaining Access

To obtain access to this database, an online application is required.[1,2] This application is instructed to be completed for any and every project you are attempting to perform with this dataset. For this data, there are some requirements. First, you must be affiliated with a Commission on Cancer (CoC)-accredited program to have access to the data. Therefore, individuals from smaller institutions may unfortunately not have ready access to this data source. Next, you will need a letter of support from the CoC-accredited cancer program on a hospital letterhead for your submitted proposal. You must also obtain a CoC Quality Portal account directly if you are the Primary Contact at your institution. Here, you will begin your official online application.

As part of this application, you will need to include the project title, principal investigator information, data analyst information, description of co-investigators, disease site, cohort of interest, primary objects, background, analysis plan, and prior experience with large datasets. Additionally, any funding will also need to be mentioned. Complete application instructions are on the application website.[2]

Converting the Files

Once you have a successful application, you will be able to download the PUFs. It is important to note that not all PUFs are the same. Depending on your application, you will get a dataset specific to the organ system of your application. For example, a brain tumor application will result in you receiving the "Brain" PUFs, while submitting a pancreatic cancer application will give you the "Pancreas" user files. Unlike the SEER database (which gives you access to every organ system once you complete the application), this database will only give you access to one type of PUF.

Additionally, once you obtain the files, you will need to convert them to a usable format. We can do this with the NCDBR package in RStudio.[3]

To do this, we can use the following code strings in the RStudio Console:

```
>install.packages("devtools")
>library(devtools)
>devtools::install_github("SophiaJia/NCDBR")
```

Once the appropriate package is downloaded, we can convert the data file using the following string:

```
>library(NCDBR)  #loads installed package NCDBR into memory
>d=getFields()   #gets wanted fields into a data frame
>d=pickFields(d)  #picks a subset of the fields and defines their types
>canc=mkNCDB(d)   #makes R binary file ~/data/NCDB/cancDef.Rdata
```

Once complete, we should be able to use our data similarly to all of the other analyses mentioned in this book. More information on converting NCDB files into an usable format and any additional package updates can be found in the online GitHub repository.[3]

Data Dictionary

The national cancer database includes more than 130 variables for each included patient. All the files can be interpreted using the PUF Data Dictionary, where you can identify what variables are included; it also lets you know the output codes for each variable and what they signify.[4]

Goals of this Dataset

The overall goal of this dataset should be to use independent variables to assess long-term overall survival attributes for patients. It can often be effective to tackle clinical research questions by using NCDB for measuring long-term outcomes and using institutional datasets for measuring short-term outcomes. When you want data on short-term outcomes and need more granular data, it is more advisable to use institutional datasets for this purpose.

Including Variables

Variables that you can include in your analysis can range widely. The dataset is effective at assessing survival outcomes with specific treatments, disparities and access to care, and measures such as treatment patterns over time. It can often be effective to research the literature for prior studies using NCDB to brainstorm ideas! Be sure to check the "PUF-VITAL_STATUS" variable in NCDB and that it is correctly coded before running statistics. In many workflows, this needs to be inverted. If not inverted for the survival algorithm, it will make your final results inaccurate. It is always a good idea to correlate your overall survival outcomes to see that they match similar previously published findings in the literature.

> Be sure to check the "PUF-VITAL_STATUS" variable in NCDB and that it is correctly coded before running statistics. In many workflows, this needs to be inverted. If not inverted for the survival algorithm, it will make your final results inaccurate. It is always a good idea to correlate your overall survival outcomes to see that they match similar previously published findings in the literature.

References

1. American College of Surgeons: Inspiring quality: Highest standards, better outcomes. Welcome to the PUF application! 2022. Accessed at: https://ncdbapp.facs.org/puf/.

2. American College of Surgeons Cancer Programs. Instructions to potential applicants. January, 2023. Accessed at: https://www.facs.org/media/xtvknrsu/2020-puf-instructions-to-potential-applicants.pdf.

3. SophiaJia. NCDBR GitHub repository. 2019. Accessed at: https://github.com/SophiaJia/NCDBR.

4. American College of Surgeons Cancer Programs. Data dictionary. September, 2023. Accessed at: https://www.facs.org/media/ujjlhni4/puf-2021-data-dictionary.pdf.

10 National Surgical Quality Improvement Database

One of the more original databases for reporting patient outcomes was the National Surgical Quality Improvement Database, also known as NSQIP. This database has origins all the way back to 1994 when the Veterans Affairs was studying complication rates in Veterans Affairs medical centers. The result of this investigation was a National Veterans Affairs Surgical Risk study from 1991 to 1993, and, subsequently, a database made available in 1994.[1] Due to this entire effort, the Veterans Affairs Hospitals reduced complications, with almost a 47% and 43% drop in mortality and morbidity rates, respectively.[1]

Later, the American College of Surgeons adopted the database and expanded it to private sector hospitals, where it is now still being employed to date.

Obtaining Access

Obtaining access to this database requires your institution to be an accredited member of the American College of Surgeons. If you attend an institution where this is the case, you can access this data through the American College of Surgeons NSQIP Portal. You will need to apply for an account, which can be found on the online application system.[2] Here, you will complete an application requesting details of your institutional affiliation, role at the institution, and also baseline demographic information. Once submitted, it will take about one week to receive a response and obtain access to the portal. Additionally, similar to the National Cancer Database, granular participant user files can also be retrieved from the American College of Surgeons for a more complete analysis and more granular data. This can be applied for and requested online.[3]

Data Stored in the Database

This database focuses on a large number of surgical procedures and hospital encounters. It contains information with respect to vascular surgery, urology, general surgery, and many others. This is data compiled across multiple different hospitals that are members of the American College of Surgeons.

This dataset is particularly useful in assessing outcomes after surgical procedures, as every patient is described with a CPT code that is relative to the principal operative procedure. Additional available variables include patient demographics, such as race, gender, and ethnicity, and hospital attributes, such as year of admission and type of operation. Unlike the larger national cancer databases, NSQIP provides more granular information, such as whether a patient is ventilator dependent, has ascites, has hypertension, specific labs, ASA classifications, wound classifications, number of pneumonia cases, reoperations, readmissions, clostridium difficile infections, and post-operative transfusion amounts. Additionally, and unlike the larger cancer databases, NSQIP only tracks mortality up to 30 days post-operation. A complete and annotated list of tracked variables by the database can be found in the participant user files dictionary.[4]

Goals for this Dataset

When compared to the larger national cancer databases, the NSQIP database is better utilized to track operative complications. For example, if there is a new procedure that is becoming widely used, assessing for complications after this procedure and comparing it to previous procedures would be helpful. Additionally, comparing perioperative complications with respect to demographics, frailty, and socioeconomic status could also be helpful.

References

1. American College of Surgeons. History. Accessed at: https://www.facs.org/quality-programs/data-and-registries/acs-nsqip/history/#:~:text=1994,rates%20from%201991%20to%202006.

2. American College of Surgeons. Application. Accessed at: https://accreditation.facs.org/programs/NSQIP.

3. American College of Surgeons. Quality programs: ACS NSQIP participant use data file. Accessed at: https://www.facs.org/quality-programs/data-and-registries/acs-nsqip/participant-use-data-file/.

4. American College of Surgeons. User guide for the 2023 ACS NSQIP Participant Use Data File (PUF). November, 2024. Accessed at: https://www.facs.org/media/ekmnc2ge/nsqip_puf_userguide_2023.pdf.

11 ClinicalTrials.gov

Another excellent data source for producing manuscripts is the ClinicalTrials.gov database, which is freely available online. In the United States, every clinical trial being performed must be registered in this database before approval for the Institutional Review Board (IRB). The National Institute of Health defines a clinical trial as:

> A research study in which one or more human subjects are prospectively assigned to one or more interventions (which may include placebo or other control) to evaluate the effects of those interventions on health-related biomedical or behavioral outcomes.[1]

This is for the purposes of tracking each study so that other investigators do not replicate the same study, to track the progress of each study since clinical trials are more long-term, and to track patient recruitment. Therefore, relevant literature exists, capturing a snapshot of all clinical trials in a particular area and summarizing them in the form of manuscripts.

Accessing the Database and Searching for Studies

The database can be freely accessed via the website.[2] Here you will find an initial search page (Fig. 11.1).

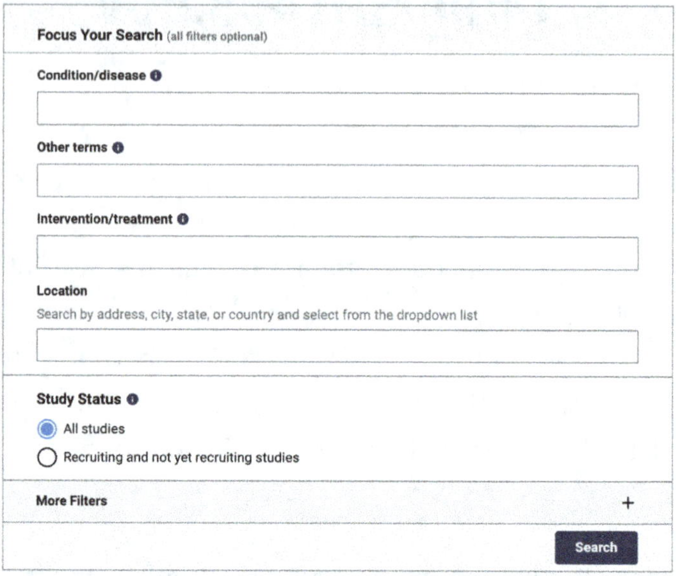

Fig. 11.1.   Initial search page of ClinicalTrials.gov.[2]

It is best to perform a search on one disease's process and an additional intervention, if possible.

Let's say we want to perform a search on diabetes mellitus type 2 and treatment with SGLT2 inhibitors. We should type "Diabetes Mellitus Type 2" in the condition/disease input and "SGLT2 inhibitor" in the intervention and treatment. As of the search in 2024, this retrieves 663 studies that we can utilize for our study. Using the left sidebars, we can further narrow down our search to those that are recruiting, not yet recruiting, active, completed, terminated, and withdrawn.

Essentially, we can create a flow chart similar to the one shown (Fig. 11.2). We can also label all exclusion criteria and how many studies were excluded per each exclusion criterion. This will make it very clear for the reader.

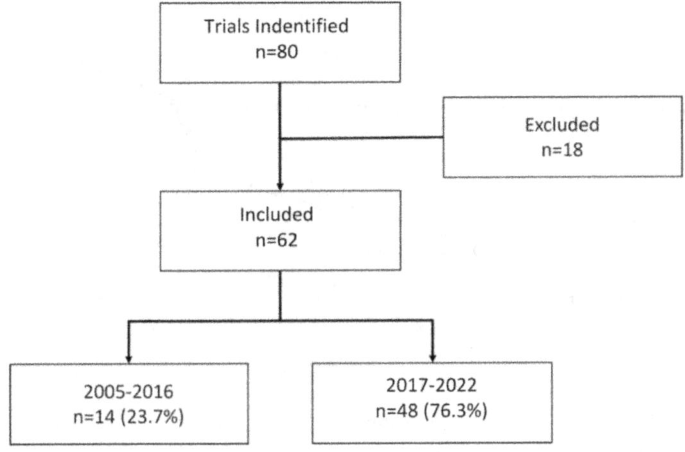

Fig. 11.2.   Flow chart depicting the selection criteria of clinical trials.

Results

Finally, once the studies are selected, it is good to clarify each study based on treatment modality. You can create bar charts stratifying each clinical trial and summarizing key components, such as treatment modality, country of origin of the study, study sample size numbers, and study status. This will make it easier for the reader to read (Fig. 11.3).

Statistics

Finally, after tabulating key statistics of each study type, you can also assess for trends in the studies using statistical tests. Common tests for these types of studies are Pearson's correlation coefficient tests to identify trends temporally over time. For example, you can identify whether there is an increasing number of studies over time versus a decrease in studies over time (Fig. 11.4).

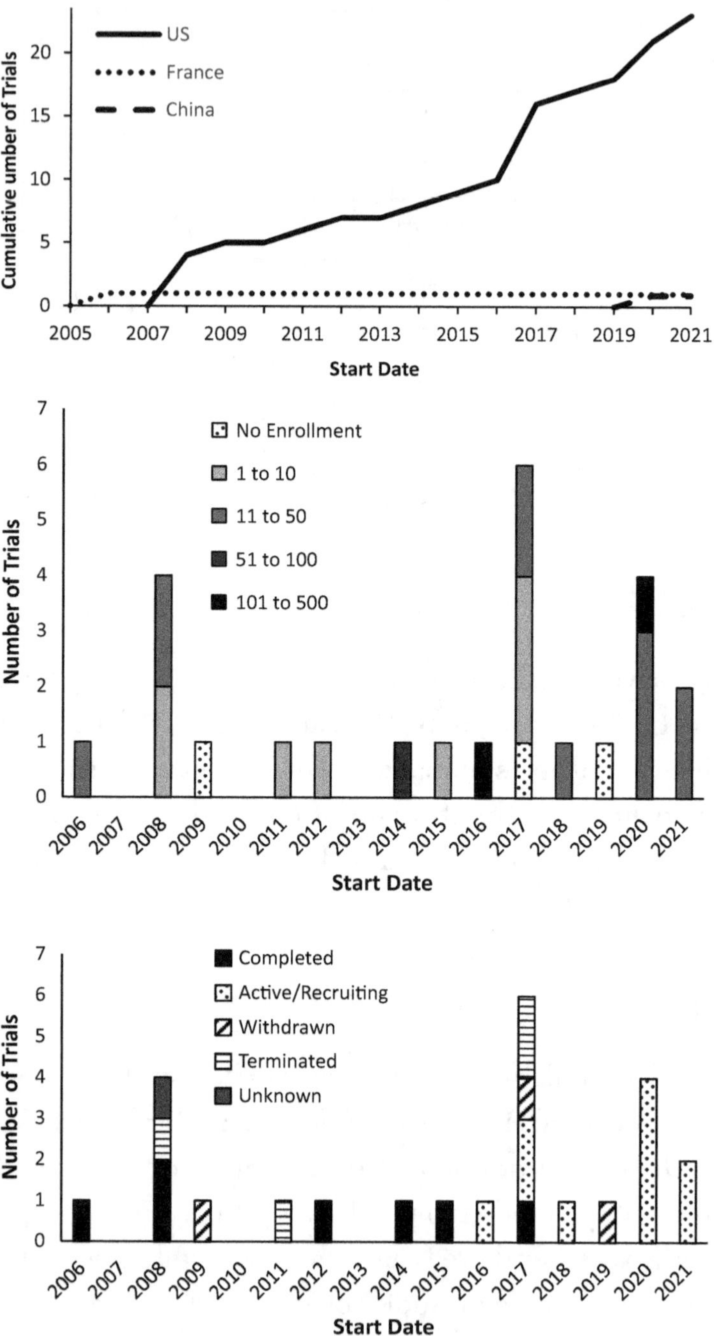

Fig. 11.3.   Bar charts depicting tabulated statistics.

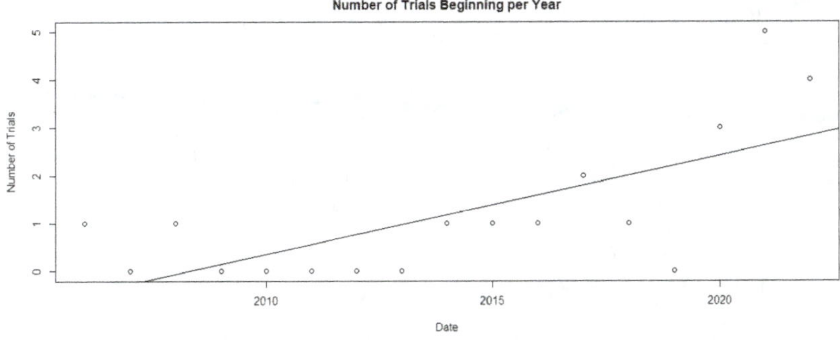

Fig. 11.4.   Uptrending number of clinical trials over time.

The correlation testing can be easily performed in RStudio using the following string:

```
>Correlationtest <- cor(Year, Number of Studies, method = "pearson")
```

Which will give you an output similar to the following:

```
data: x and y
t = 1.4186, df = 5, p-value = 0.2152
alternative hypothesis: true correlation is not equal to 0
95 percent confidence interval:
 -0.3643187     0.9183058
sample estimates:
cor
0.5357143
```

Where the p-value is 0.2152 and the correlation coefficient (how strong the correlation is) is 0.5357.

To make categorical comparisons among the different types of clinical trials, you could use Pearson's chi-square test, which can be performed using the following RStudio string when you have your data formatted for what you want to compare:

```
test <- chisq.test(table(dat$Species, dat$size))
```

Which will lead to the following output:

```
Pearson's Chi-squared test
##
## data:  table(dat$Species, dat$size)
## X-squared = 86.035, df = 2, p-value < 2.2e-16
```

Where the p-value is <0.001 in this case.

In addition to statistical findings, it is often useful to categorize preliminary findings from studies that have published results on the website. On the website, you will find any reported adverse events and preliminary data reported by the investigators. Additionally, another good aspect to add to your manuscript is to search each included clinical trial number on PubMed (begins with NCT and is 8 digits in length) and provide references for completed studies that already have completely published data. Doing all of these tasks included in this chapter will help you successfully publish a manuscript using this database.

Overall, points to discuss would include which clinical trials have already been completed and what the results of these clinical trials are. What are the current clinical trials that are recruiting at this time? Is there an area of this treatment modality that is not currently well investigated by those currently listed on ClinicalTrials.gov?

Conclusion

Performing studies using the ClinicalTrials.gov database can be an invaluable method for characterizing the current state of clinical trials for a new treatment modality for diseases. These types of papers can provide insight into what are being performed, preliminary results, and clinical trials that may need to be carried out in the future.

References

1. National Institutes of Health Grants & Funding. NIH's definition of a clinical trial. September 18, 2024. Accessed at: https://grants.nih.gov/policy/clinical-trials/definition.htm.
2. National Library of Medicine: National Center for Biotechnology Information. Focus your search. Accessed at: https://clinicaltrials.gov.

12 Manufacturer and User Facility Device Experience Database

One excellent resource that is available to use is the Manufacturer and User Facility Device Experience (MAUDE) database. Supported by the United States Food and Drug Administration (FDA), the MAUDE database offers a repository of adverse events for all medical devices approved by the FDA in the United States. As part of the clinical trial process, Phase 4 constitutes the post-approval surveillance of devices, and this database acts as a repository of adverse events for each FDA-approved device.

Every medical device approved by and in use in the United States is available in this database. Best of all, this database is free of charge and publicly available without requiring any credentials to assess this data. This database is an excellent resource to use for characterizing adverse events and areas of improvement for medical devices. Here, we will discuss how to use this data in writing your manuscript.

Initial Search

This database can be easily accessed online by anyone with Internet access.[1] Here, you will find many search fields to assess the model and problem that you would like. Overall, it is ideally best to narrow down both by device type and also by brand if possible. This may be the easiest to perform with devices that have a high number of entries, such as orthotics or interventional cardiology devices, but some more specialized devices may not have enough entries to perform an entire study by themselves. In these cases, you could consider having descriptive characteristics for one device but different types of brands.

Once narrowed down by device and, ideally, brand, you can initially stratify your search using the "product problem" search term to identify all problems of a particular type. You can even stratify for an injury that occurred versus death. You can also specify the search timeframe that you would like to use. Keep in mind that when you tune your search parameters, the database will only intrinsically populate 500 items at a time. Therefore, to obtain longer timeframes, you would need to strategically finetune your search to include dates that only result in <500 items at a time and then add them all together at the end into one larger spreadsheet.

Once you hit "search," a list of adverse events will populate the webpage with lists of ten entries each. In most cases, it is better to click "Export to Excel" in the top right corner to produce this into a user-friendlier Excel file.

Data Extraction

Once in the Excel file, you will have a user-friendly list of all device-related complications. Unfortunately, due to the unstandardized nature of this data, an investigator often has to search the data and organize it effectively. Duplicate entries may be used in the database for one adverse event. Therefore, it is best to sort your Excel spreadsheet by adverse event date and also by report number. If multiple entries are entered on the same adverse event, these can be compiled, and duplicates can be removed. This can often happen when an adverse event occurs, both the hospital and the patient report the incident to the FDA.

There can be many duplicate entries filed in this database. Therefore, it is extremely important to screen for these duplicate entries before performing any analysis or assessment.

The Excel spreadsheet will have the following headings (Table 12.1):

Table 12.1.   Variables Found in the MAUDE Database

Variable	Relevance
Web address	Direct link to the individual report
Report number	Unique identifying report number — this should be used to remove duplicate entries during your data extraction process
Event date	Date the event occurred — this can also be used to help identify duplicate events
Event type	Generally dichotomized to injury versus malfunction, sometimes will be death
Manufacturer	The entity that produced the device
Date received	Date the report was received
Brand name	Brand name for the device
Device problem	Categorical description of the event
Patient problem	Effects the adverse event had on the patient
PMA/PMN number	FDA premarket approval number
Exemption number	FDA exemption number
Number of events	Number of reported events
Event text	Complete narrative description of adverse event

Creating a Manuscript

We can only comment on the rates of adverse events as a proportion; therefore, pie charts can be utilized to describe which adverse events occur more than other events. Of note, sometimes reaching out to device representatives will allow the representatives to produce a quote on how many devices were used during the time period searched in your study.

This can give you an estimation of the prevalence of adverse events over this timeframe:

$$\frac{\text{Number of adverse events reports in the database}}{\text{Number of events estimated by representative}}$$

Additionally, we can also characterize if any deaths or serious bodily injury occurred with these devices. These are all pertinent questions that can be answered by this data for new devices that have been in development for <10 years but have little published data. Finally, the written entry portions of the data can be summarized to provide recommendations to manufacturers, and this can be provided in a manuscript format.

Limitations

Unfortunately, several limitations exist with this database. The number of devices currently used in the United States of that particular type is not provided in the database. Therefore, no statements can be made on the prevalence of adverse events unless a representative is willing to provide you with an estimate of the number of devices used. If they are unwilling, or you are unable to get in contact with one, estimating the prevalence of adverse events will not be feasible.

Another common limitation of this dataset is that manufacturers are required to report adverse events; however, patients may also report adverse device events to the FDA, thus making duplicate entries, as previously discussed:

In accordance with 21 CFR Part 803, manufacturers and importers must submit reports when they become aware of information that reasonably suggests that one of their marketed devices may have caused or contributed to a death or serious injury or has malfunctioned, and the malfunction of the device or a similar device that they market would be likely to cause or contribute to a death or serious injury if the malfunction were to recur.[2] Manufacturers must send reports of such deaths, serious injuries, and malfunctions to the FDA. Importers must send reports of deaths and serious injuries to the FDA and the manufacturer and reports of malfunctions to the manufacturer.[2]

Device user facilities include hospitals, outpatient diagnostic or treatment facilities, nursing homes, and ambulatory surgical facilities. Device user facilities must submit reports when they become aware of information that reasonably suggests that a device may have caused or contributed to a death or serious injury of a patient in their facility. Death reports must be sent to the FDA and the manufacturer if known. Serious injury reports must be sent to the manufacturer or the FDA if the manufacturer is not known.[2]

Therefore, what can happen is that the manufacturer reports an event while the patient reports the same event to the FDA. This will create duplicate entries for the same event. If possible, it is advised to go and screen these as much as possible when extracting data.

Additionally, just because an adverse event is reported to the MAUDE database, it does not mean it is verified that it has totally occurred. The following US Code reflects this issue.

Section 21 CFR 803.16 states that "A report or other information submitted by a reporting entity under this part, and any release by FDA of that report or information, does not necessarily reflect a conclusion by the party submitting the report or by FDA that the report or information constitutes an admission that the device, or the reporting entity or its employees, caused or contributed to the reportable event. The reporting entity need not admit and may deny that the report or information submitted under this part constitutes an admission that the device, the party submitting the report, or employees thereof, caused or contributed to a reportable event."[3]

Conclusions

Overall, the MAUDE database has many limitations; however, it is a valuable tool in addressing some aspects of newly approved medical devices and is used by the United States for device surveillance. Typical manuscripts using this database would capture the proportion of adverse events reported for a typical device of a single brand and estimate adverse event prevalence, if possible.

References

1. United States Food & Drug Administration. Manufacturer and user facility device experience database. December 21, 2024. Accessed at: https://www.accessdata.fda.gov/scripts/cdrh/cfdocs/cfmaude/search.cfm.
2. National Archives. Code of federal regulations. December 9, 2024. Accessed at: https://www.ecfr.gov/current/title-21/chapter-I/subchapter-H/part-803.
3. National Archives. Code of federal regulations. December 18, 2024. Accessed at: https://www.ecfr.gov/current/title-21/chapter-I/subchapter-H/part-803/subpart-A/section-803.16.

13 MarketScan Database

When you are attempting to assess variables such as diagnosis codes, prescription fills, and insurance information among patients, a large national database can be used known as the MarketScan Database.[1] Created by IBM, this database has information on over 250 million patients across the United States, and it has several unique variables that are not easily identified using other datasets. One of the disadvantages is the difficulty in accessing this database and the learning curve for utilizing its data. It is a database limited to specific institutions. However, if you are able to successfully complete the learning curve, it offers plenty of data not available from other resources.

Unique Variables

This dataset is able to provide information on insurance type, lab results, outpatient drug information, and inpatient drug usage and information. These are all variables not easily assessed by other national databases and are a strength of this dataset. There is also focused information on hospital discharges and information from patient discharge to inpatient rehabilitation and skilled nursing facilities.[2] Dental information is also stored in these datasets.[2]

Obtaining Access

Access to this database is generally institution-specific, with an office of institutional research approving access. This dataset often comes with a small fee associated with the dataset and can be viewed from an online portal.[3] If you do not have institutional access to this database, an applicant can apply directly to IBM for access to this dataset; however, it is more difficult this way.

Limitations

One significant limitation of this dataset is the limited availability and often-lengthy processing times for obtaining access. Requests for access can take >6 months for individuals without local institutional access already in place. Additionally, even with local and institutional access, there is sometimes a small fee for access to the sample.

References

1. Watson Health. Welcome to MarketScan Research. 2018. Accessed at: https://www.ibm.com/watson/health/resources/ipv-opv/.
2. Stanford Medicine: Center for Population Health Sciences. 2024. Accessed at: https://med.stanford.edu/phs/data/marketscan-data.html.
3. Stanford University. MarketScan databases. 2024. Accessed at: https://redivis.com/datasets/96hs-egqe74693.

14 Nationwide Readmissions Database

If you are attempting to assess the number of readmissions among individuals being discharged from the hospital, the Nationwide Readmissions Database is a good resource.[1] The Nationwide Readmissions Database (otherwise known as NRD) was a database originally developed for the Healthcare Cost and Utilization Project (HCUP).[1] It primarily focuses on readmissions of all ages and was focused on being the first nationally representative model of its kind.

Without using the dataset weights, it contains roughly 16.8 million discharges; however, it contains approximately 33.4 million patient information otherwises.[1] These weights can be implemented using statistical processing software such as RStudio to make a higher overall n-value. It was intended to be a platform to make decisions on the national, state, and community levels.

Using the Dataset

The dataset can be used in two different commonly used formats. The first is an individual-level format, where the patients are identified by ICD-10-CM diagnosis codes. From here, the researcher can identify any comorbidity and readmission occurred by the patient.[1] A second set of data can be identified with hospital-level files that contain characteristics on a hospital level.[1]

Unique Variables

Unique variables provided by this dataset include the ability to assess readmissions over a long period of time. While being primarily identified via ICD-10-CM diagnoses codes, the researcher can identify both short- and long-term readmissions data, which is commonly not found in other datasets.[1] Additionally, it has information on costs associated with readmissions, the reason for the readmissions, and readmissions by special populations.[1]

Another important consideration of this dataset is the use of weighted information. Without the use of weights, the dataset is half of what the dataset would be with the use of weights. Therefore, this is important to consider when thinking about your statistical plan for the data in your study. There are several online resources to consult to learn about the use of weighting systems in large datasets, including the *weights* package in RStudio.[2]

Accessing the Datasets

The Nationwide Readmission Dataset is publicly available through a data use agreement.[1] Many institutions likely have existing agreements that researchers can use to access the data. However, if your institution does not have access, one would need to be developed and applied to have access.

References

1. Agency for Healthcare Research and Quality. HCUP-US overview. Accessed at: https://hcup-us.ahrq.gov/nrdoverview.jsp.
2. The Comprehensive R Archive Network. Package 'weights'. October 12, 2022. Accessed at: https://cran.r-project.org/web/packages/weights/weights.pdf.

15 Global Burden of Disease Database

The Global Burden of Disease Database is an outstanding resource used to assess medical statistics for a wide variety of diseases internationally. Developed by the Institute for Health Metrics and Evaluation at the University of Washington in 2021, they published the Global Burden of Diseases, Injuries, and Risk Factors Study, which uses 328,938 data sources and reveals health disparities across age, sex, locations, and socioeconomic groups.[1] As a result of this study, all of this global data was made public and available for download so that other researchers could use this data. For clinical researchers, this is one of the only database resources for international data.

Accessing the Data

Much of this information is available and free for use online.[2] However, individuals will need to make an account with the Institute for Health Metrics and Evaluation (IHME). Creating an account is a short process requiring the user to get an online profile, complete a small course on epidemiology, and have the account approved by IHME. Once this is complete, you can access all of the data available.

Captured Data Points

This is an important database to study diseases globally, a key factor missing from other commonly used databases in clinical research. In this database, you can assess many epidemiological metrics that are not offered in any other databases.[2] A listing of some of these metrics is provided in Table 15.1:

The database contains a large amount of information to pull from and includes several forecast datasets. This includes datasets for smoking mortality and prevalence forecasts, lead exposure estimates, disability weights, years lived with disability, disability-adjusted life years and healthy life, and many more available forecasts.

To assess the data, the IHME provides a set of eight different tools for use. This includes the GBD Results Tool, GBD Compare, GBD Foresight, Mortality Visualization (MortViz), Causes of Death Visualization (CoDViz), Epi Visualization (EpiViz), Burden of Proof Visualization (BoPViz), and GBD Sources Tool.[3]

Table 15.1. Table of Epidemiological Metrics Assessed by the Global Burden of Disease Database[2]

Metric	Description
Disability-adjusted life years (DALYs)	Years of healthy life lost to premature death and disability
Healthy life expectancy	The number of years that a person at a given age can expect to live in good health, taking into account mortality and disability
Years lived with disability (YLDs)	Years of life lived with any short-term or long-term health loss
Years of life lost (YLLs)	Years of life lost due to premature mortality
Life expectancy	Number of years a person is expected to live based on their present age

Dataset Ideas

Many different ideas can be pursued using this dataset. Examples include estimating the forecasted prevalence of diseases in the future to include the variables mentioned in Table 15.1. Additionally, ideas can include evaluating changes in disease prevalence over the most recent decades and identifying areas that need more targeted interventions.

Global Burden of Disease Collaborator Network

Currently, the Global Burden of Disease Collaborator Network is seeking collaborators to make meaningful contributions to the Global Burden of Disease affiliated studies.[4] This process would consist of applying to the Collaborator Network, taking a small course on epidemiological principles, and then getting invited to review and make meaningful contributions to future studies using the Global Burden of Disease Database. The call for collaborators is for all individuals in all aspects and interests in medicine; however, collaborators only typically review manuscripts/studies that are relevant to their field of expertise. Applications can be prepared and submitted online.[5]

Participating in this collaboration is an excellent way to become involved with epidemiology and make meaningful contributions to the literature.

References

1. Institute for Health Metrics and Evaluation. Global Burden of Disease 2021: Findings from the GBD 2021 Study. 2024. Accessed at: https://www.healthdata.org/sites/default/files/2024-05/GBD_2021_Booklet_FINAL_2024.05.16.pdf.

2. Institute for Health Metrics and Evaluation. Global Burden of Disease Study 2021 (GBD 2021) data resources. 2024. Accessed at: https://ghdx.healthdata.org/gbd-2021.

3. Institute for Health Metrics and Evaluation. GBD data and tools guide. Accessed at: https://www.healthdata.org/research-analysis/about-gbd/gbd-data-and-tools-guide.

4. Institute for Health Metrics and Evaluation. GBD collaborator network. https://www.healthdata.org/research-analysis/gbd/collaborator-network#call.

5. Institute for Health Metrics and Evaluation. Application for collaborator. 2024. Accessed at: https://gbdcollaboratorportal.healthdata.org/aspx/application.

16 TriNetX Database

The TriNetX database is a novel database that was designed in 2013.[1] It was designed by a for-profit company named TriNetX with the goal of making a database that was user-friendly, on-demand, and able to be used by global and diverse populations. They also wanted a database that could easily reuse information from electronic health records and be versatile.[1] The original purpose was to allow pharmaceutical companies and other industry partners to find institutions that would be good clinical sites for launching clinical trials and other tests.[1]

Accessing the Data

This database is available via an online portal for researchers.[2] Typically, a researcher would need to be at an institution that participates in the TriNetX database. Therefore, if you are not at a participating institution, it may be difficult to access this dataset. Once you create an institutional account, it is typically free for use for most researchers. Otherwise, it is typically available at a small fee to obtain access to the online portal system.[3,4] Once you have an institutional account, access to the data can be found online via a login website.[3]

Types of Data

Even though multiple institutions are involved with TriNetX, users can typically only see local data from their own institution.[1] A limited number of institutions can query data from other institutions. This novel dataset integrates with electronic health records across multiple institutions and is being continuously updated to consist of more recent data than other databases mentioned in this book.

It is unique in that it also consists of a wide variety of data from hospital in-patients and primary care and specialty treatment providers. It also has information on demographics, insurance, services, medications, medical conditions, labs, clinical observations, and genomic information.[3] It also contains international data from institutions across 30 different countries.[3]

Search Criteria

Search criteria are generally performed via disease name or patient CPT codes,[5] whereas exclusion criteria can be performed using disease names and CPT codes. Additional search ranges can also be performed with basic demographics. An excellent example video of performing a TriNetX database query can be found online.[5]

Analytics

Lastly, this is one of the only databases that allow you to perform data analytics online through the database platform. This database allows researchers to compare outcomes with basic regression, propensity score matching, and other statistical methods with their online and easy-to-use user-friendly interface portal. This has the additional advantage of making the data extraction and statistical analysis project more efficient. As more and more institutions enroll in this novel database, access to continuously updated information will allow individuals greater access to up-to-date data to use for clinical outcomes studies.

References

1. TriNetX. About us. 2022. Accessed at: https://trinetx.com/about-trinetx/.
2. TriNetX. TriNetX. 2024. Accessed at: https://live.trinetx.com.
3. TriNetX. TriNetX datasets. 2022. Accessed at: https://trinetx.com/solutions/real-world-datasets/#s_4.
4. MaineHealth. TriNetX. 2017. Accessed at: https://mhir.org/?page_id=42633#:~:text=Security%3A%20TriNetX%20is%20fully%20HIPAA,%2Didentified%20queries%2Fcohort%20development.
5. WFBMI Host. TriNetX — A brief overview. 2021. Accessed at: https://www.youtube.com/watch?v=T7qpxjaK9z4.

17 Centers for Medicare and Medicaid Services Part B National Summary Data File

The Centers for Medicare and Medicaid Services maintains a database that includes prices and a number of procedures for all CPT-related procedural and service codes conducted in the United States that are reimbursed by Medicare and Medicaid services. This can be accessed for free online.[1] It contains data from 2000 to 2021 by the time of this writing.

This database is one of the only unique databases that look at the cost of each procedure or service. Therefore, it is a great resource to use when attempting to compare the outcomes of different types of procedural treatments, such as in Table 17.1.

You can also use this resource to compare treatment procedure volumes that are billed to either Medicare or Medicaid, such as in Fig. 17.1.

Table 17.1. Differences in Annual Procedure Volume Before and After 2015

Procedure	Pre-2015 volume (Mean ± SD)	Post-2015 volume (Mean ± SD)	P-value
Exploratory craniotomy	387.13 ± 65.3	528.43 ± 21.2	0.00002
Craniotomy for abscess	349.53 ± 63.3	496.86 ± 33.8	0.00001
Craniotomy for AVM	121.07 ± 11.8	141.86 ± 18.0	0.004

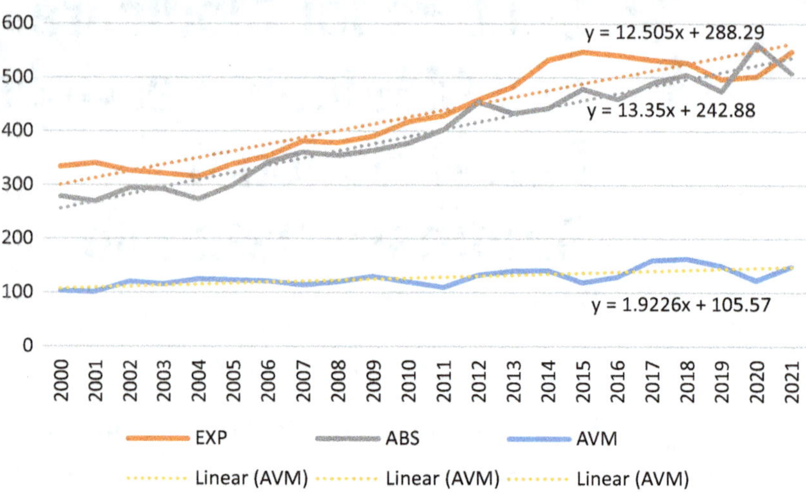

Fig. 17.1.   Comparison of the annual volume of procedures billed to Medicare Type B each year for exploratory craniotomy (EXP), craniotomy for abscess (ABS), and craniotomy for AVM (AVM).

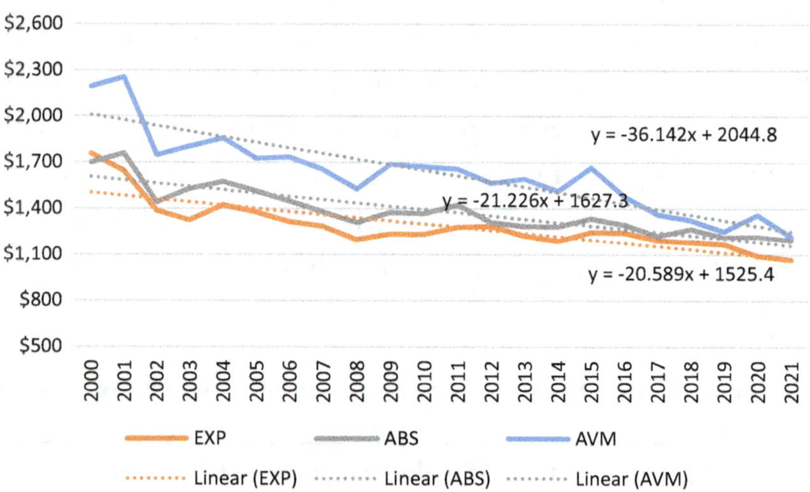

Fig. 17.2.   Comparison of inflation-adjusted Mean Medicare reimbursement to physicians per exploratory craniotomy (EXP), craniotomy for abscess (ABS), and craniotomy for AVM (AVM).

Finally, in your study, you can also adjust for inflation on a yearly basis to have an updated cost comparison. For example, reimbursement may appear to be increasing over time, but if you adjust for inflation, you may see that the treatment reimbursement is actually decreasing when inflation is adjusted.

Reference

1. Centers for Medicare & Medicaid Services. Part B National summary data file (Previously known as BESS). September 10, 2024. Accessed at: https://www.cms.gov/data-research/statistics-trends-and-reports/part-b-national-summary-data-file.

Part IV
Data Analysis

18 Bivariable and Multivariable Comparisons

Now that you have gathered your data, it is time to perform statistical analysis. This book does not suggest you should perform these analyses without any assistence from a statistician — it is simply meant to be an adjunct to learning to perform these analyses yourself. It is very important that before you submit your work for publication, you have all of your analyses evaluated by a person with a formal statistics background.

That being said, in this chapter, we will educate you on how to perform simple statistical comparisons using both bivariable and multivariable models using RStudio.

RStudio

In this book, we will solely discuss statistics in RStudio. There are a few reasons for this choice.[1] First, RStudio is free for download, while other programs may charge hefty fees for downloading their statistical software. Second, RStudio is open-source and supports commercial usage. Therefore, you are free to do whatever you would like with your results from RStudio. Finally, much of the data analysis with respect to clinical outcomes right now, at the time of this writing, is being performed with RStudio; thus, if you need any assistance or example scripts to help you perform your coding, it would be of your best interest to perform this in RStudio. You always, generally speaking, want to use the same programs that experts in your field are using so that you do not have to reinvent the wheel with something someone else has already discovered. For all these reasons, RStudio is ideal for medical students and other junior healthcare professionals.

The first task is to download RStudio, which is available for both Windows and Mac and can be found here.[1] This can be easily installed by using the prompts after downloading. Once downloaded and opened, it will look something like Fig. 18.1. At marker **A**, this is where we will save previously created R scripts. At **B**, this is where RStudio will store your R script history. At **C**, this is where we will find your console where you can write scripts. Finally, at **D**, this is where the output of your codes will be displayed. First, we want to upload your data, which will likely be in an Excel spreadsheet.

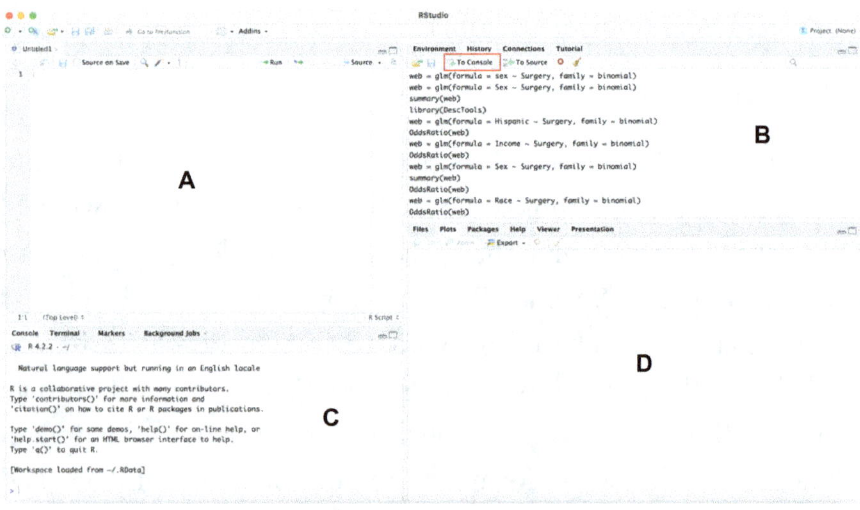

Fig. 18.1.   Initial RStudio workstation.[1]

Cleaning the Data and Upload

Before you get started, you will want to clean your data. If you get your data from an institutional local dataset, or if you obtain your data from a national database, a typical format would be to store the data in a Microsoft Excel format. Therefore, you would have one patient for each row and have columns for your variables. "Cleaning" the data refers to setting your data up for statistical analysis. Therefore, we need to make several changes.

To process our data, we need to change all wording in the Excel spreadsheet to numerals. Dichotomous variables such as sex should be changed from "male" or "female" to "1" or "0." Likewise, Hispanic should be changed from "Hispanic" or "non-Hispanic" to "1" or "0." Additionally, all continuous variables should be strictly numeric only. Instead of cells containing words with numbers such as "56 years of age," we need to change this to "56." These changes can commonly be performed using Microsoft Excel and clicking "Edit" and "Find" and "Find and Replace" — this will allow you to directly replace any wording in all cells once the cells are highlighted. Essentially, there should be no letters in your Excel document once completed.

> There are many ways to clean data inclusive of script writing once the data is actually uploaded into RStudio. For simplicity here, we only discuss making modifications in Microsoft Excel.

Once complete, your Excel spreadsheet is ready to be uploaded into RStudio. Click the red box in Fig. 18.1. If done successfully, you should then see the following code input in your workstation.

```
>NCDB_Tumors <-
read_excel("C:/Users/tanma/OneDrive/Desktop/NCDB_
Tumors.xlsx")
```

Additionally, you will also need to "attach" your data using the following script. This sets up your data to run code in RStudio:

```
>attach(NCDB_Tumors)
```

Chi-Square Tests (Categorical Comparisons)

To perform initial chi-squared tests for categorical comparisons among baseline cohorts, you would need to download and install the *stats* package:

```
>Install.packages(stats)
```

Once you download a package, you will also need to library the package for each use using the following code:

```
>library(stats)
```

Once this package is libraried and your data is attached, you can make chi-squared comparisons using the *stats* package. Here is an example code string using the NCDB_Tumor dataset and comparing an independent categorical variable ("treatment") and assessing the dependent outcome variable ("improvement").

```
>chisq.test(NCDB_Tumor$treatment, NCDB_Tumor$improvement,
correct=FALSE)
```

The following output would be:

```
            Pearson's Chi-squared test
data: NCDB_Tumor$treatment and NCDB_Tumor$improvement
X-squared = 2.3069, df = 1, p-value = 0.03456
```

Student' t-tests

This can be performed innately in RStudio using the following formula:

```
>t.test(NCDB_Tumor$treatment~ NCDB_Tumor$improvement,
data=NCDB_Tumor)
```

Where x is a numeric vector or a column from the data and y is a binary variable separating the groups. The output will look similar to this:

```
Welch Two Sample t-test

data:  Income by Sex
t = 0.49396, df = 64580, p-value = 0.6213
alternative hypothesis: true difference in means between group 1 and
group 2 is not equal to 0
95 percent confidence interval:
 -0.009326711  0.015611719
sample estimates:
mean in group 1 mean in group 2
     3.017067       3.013924
```

With this information showing not significant results due to the p-value = 0.6213.

Logistic and Linear Regression

The first types of algorithms we will discuss are the simple logistic regression and linear regressions, which will be performed using the "glm" function. This would take the following format as a formula in the console:

```
>glm(formula = Age ~ `Improvement`)
```

Where we are comparing the relationship of symptom improvement with respect to age. Performing this results in the following:

```
Deviance Residuals:
   Min      1Q  Median     3Q     Max
-44.269 -14.919   1.081  16.081  51.081

Coefficients:
                Estimate Std. Error t value Pr(>|t|)
(Intercept)        45.019      2.464  18.273  <2e-16 ***
`Improvement`      -5.100      2.582  -1.976  0.0486 *
---
Signif. codes:  0 '***' 0.001 '**' 0.01 '*' 0.05 '.' 0.1 ' ' 1

(Dispersion parameter for gaussian family taken to be 430.9558)

Null deviance: 343861 on 795 degrees of freedom
Residual deviance: 342179 on 794 degrees of freedom

(57 observations deleted due to missingness)
AIC: 7091.5

Number of Fisher Scoring iterations: 2
```

Here, we can see that our estimate is −5.100. Overall, this means that with increasing age, a patient is less likely to have symptom improvement. Additionally, this finding is significant, as we can see with a p-value of $p = 0.0486$.

Here is how we can turn this into an odds ratio that is easier to be read and placed in tables for manuscripts. First, we need to install a new package named DescTools. This can be done with activating the following code.

```
>Install.packages(DescTools)
```

After the installation, we will additionally need to add it to our RStudio library every time we use it.

```
>library(DescTools)
```

Next, we can save our previous linear regression run to a useable model.

```
>Symptoms <- glm(formula = Age ~ `Improvement`)
```

Then, we can perform odds ration on our model.

```
>OddsRatio(Symptoms)
```

This will result in the following output.

```
Call:
glm(formula = Age ~ Improvement)

Odds Ratios:
                              or or.lci or.uci Pr(>|z|)
(Intercept)                5.799 1.740 19.329 0.0042 **
Symptom Improvement        0.985 0.980 0.990 0.0486 ***

Signif. codes: 0 ***** 0.001 **** 0.01 *** 0.05 '.' 0.1 ' * 1
Brier Score: 0.137          Nagelkerke RZ: 0.048
```

This is where we can see that our odds ratio for symptom improvement for increasing age is 0.985 with a confidence interval of 0.980–0.990. The p-value associated with this assessment is 0.0486.

Since we were only assessing associations between one variable and another variable directly, this would be termed a bivariable association. To perform a multivariable logistic regression, we would follow a similar process; however, we would essentially just add additional variables to the strings. Here is an example of a more complex multivariable assessment with more variables added:

```
>Symptoms <- glm(formula = Surgery_Recommended ~ Age + Sex + Race + Ethnicity +Marital_Status_Group + Total_Tumors + Median_Household_Income_Group +Rural_Urban)
```

When going through the following steps as above, the following string results:

```
Call:
glm(formula = Surgery_Recommended ~ Age + Sex + Race +
Ethnicity + Marital_Status_Group + Total_Tumors + Median_Household_
Income_Group + Rural_Urban, family = binomial, data = cleaned_
data)
```

Odds Ratios:	or	or.lci	or.uci	Pr(>|z|)
(Intercept)	5.799	1.740	19.329	0.0042 **
Age	0.985	0.980	0.990	1.38e-08 ***
SexMale	1.072	0.866	1.326	0.5257
RaceAsian or Pacific Islander	1.634	0.498	5.359	0.4181
RaceBlack	1.500	0.467	4.816	0.4958
RaceWhite	1.679	0.534	5.279	0.3750
EthnicitySpanish-Hispanic-Latino	1.350	0.996	1.830	0.0532
Marital_Status_GroupMarried	1.684	1.319	2.151	2.93e-05 ***
Total_Tumors	0.692	0.560	0.855	6.54e-04 ***
Median_Household_Income_Group>= $75,000	1.032	0.821	1.298	0.7865
Rural_UrbanUrban	1.088	0.772	1.531	0.6307

```
Signif. codes: 0 ***** 0.001 **** 0.01 *** 0.05 '.' 0.1 ' ' * 1
Brier Score: 0.137                    Nagelkerke RZ: 0.048
```

Here, we have the resulting odds ratios and confidence interval, each adjusted variable, along with p-values for each variable.

Assessing Model Accuracy

To check the accuracy of our model, we generally check the area under the curve, otherwise known as AUC. See Fig. 18.2.

This is where we have the true positive rate on the y-axis and the false positive rate on the x-axis. Here, we are attempting to maximize the area under the curve where this area ranges from 0 to 1.0. In practicality, virtually no model achieves 1.0, which is a perfect model. However, there is a set of guidelines that can be used for accuracy. In general, an AUC of 0.5 suggests no discrimination (i.e., ability to diagnose patients with and without the disease or condition based on the test), 0.7 to 0.8 is considered acceptable, 0.8 to 0.9 is considered excellent, and more than 0.9

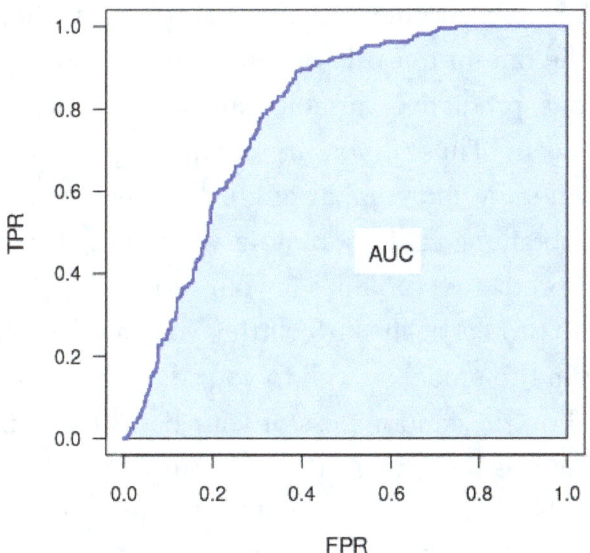

Fig. 18.2.   Area under the curve (AUC).[2]

is considered outstanding.[3] Generally speaking, in medical literature, a model is acceptable over the 0.70 threshold.

This can be performed by installing the DescTools package:

```
>install.packages("DescTools")
```

Then, we must library our new package:

```
>library(DescTools)
```

Next, we perform the c-statistic:

```
>Cstat(Symptoms)
```

Which will give us the following output:

```
[1] 0.6927984
```

One in Ten Rule of Multivariable Analysis

When performing a multivariable model, it is important to
remember the one-in-ten rule of multivariable models. This rule
states that one predictive variable can be studied for every ten
events that occur. Thus, if you are comparing how many people
obtain radiotherapy and comparing this between two cohorts and
40 patients obtaining radiotherapy in your dataset, you can only
include four predictive variables in your model.

This is to protect against overfitting your model, which essentially will train the model so well to your data that it will train the
model based on the randomness of your data. This will also take
the form of an overly high c-statistic of your model, as obtained by
the method above. It is a complicated concept; however, for the
purposes of this book, just be sure to know you can only include
so many variables in your multivariable model for every ten events

being measured. If your study has 200 events being measured, you can include 20 variables in the multivariable model. If you are using national database data that includes 500,000 events, you can use as many variables as you would like.

Testing Variance Influence Factors

As the last part of our analysis, we will check variance influence factors (VIFs). In a multivariable model, two variables could be collinear with each other, and one of the collinear variables should be removed from the model. For example, you may find that obesity and diabetes could be two collinear variables, and one should be removed from the model if this occurs. Variables are generally considered to be collinear if the VIFs are >5.0. We can test this using the following formulate in RStudio, which requires the previously installed *DescTools* package:

```
>VIF(Symptoms)
```

As a result of running this command, all of the variables listed in the output should be <5.0 or removed from the analysis if >5.0.

Hosmer-Lemeshow Goodness-of-Fit Test

An additional measure of model accuracy is the goodness-of-fit test, which determines how well a linear regression model fits a set of data by comparing the overserved values to those predicted by the model.[4] This can be performed using the following code provided in the *glmtoolbox* package:

```
>hltest(Symptoms)
```

An ideal result is one with a negative p-value, indicating adequate goodness-of-fit.[5]

Publishable Findings

When making conclusions from your analyses, there are generally two types of findings that may lead to publishable data. First, findings that are statistically significant are generally publishable if they are clinically relevant. For example, if you find that one patient population has better access to care if they are a certain race for a particular disease and this is statistically significant and clinically relevant, this is generally publishable. A second type of publishable finding can take the form of non-significant findings. For example, if you find that living in a certain regional area does not make you more likely to have speedy treatment, this could be clinically relevant. In these types of null findings, however, you often need to have other variables that are statistically significant to help show the journal reviewers that your study is sufficiently powered to make this claim. If you show that living in a certain region does not have an effect on treatment outcomes and that age and income are also not significant, this can really just be due to an underpowered study. Therefore, it is often best to have null findings with other variables that are statistically significant present in the analysis.

Resource for Further Graph Ideas

For my ideas and code support with plots, check out The R Graph Gallery,[6] which includes great resources to find any figure that would be ideal for your particular manuscript. Additional resources for using the "glm" function are available at Rdocumentation.[7]

References

1. Posit. Download RStudio Desktop. November 4, 2024. Accessed at: https://posit.co/download/rstudio-desktop/.

2. ProfGigio. The area under a ROC curve. January 20, 2022. Accessed at: https://commons.wikimedia.org/wiki/File:Basic_AUC_annotated.png.

3. Hosmer DW, Lemeshow S, Sturdivant R, *et al*. Applied logistic regression. July 31, 1989. Accessed at: https://books.google.com/books?hl=en&lr=&id=bRoxQBIZRd4C&oi=fnd&pg=PR13&ots=kM2Ntn8X-b7&sig=O8trbcFJZe3Aess4DX7l-4odAyo#v=onepage&q&f=false.

4. R Package Documentation. hltest: The Hosmer-Lemeshow Goodness-of-Fit Test. September 11, 2024. Accessed at: https://rdrr.io/cran/glmtoolbox/man/hltest.html.

5. IBM. Tests of model fit. September 9, 2024. Accessed at: https://www.ibm.com/docs/en/spss-statistics/saas?topic=diagnostics-tests-model-fit.

6. R Graph Gallery. The R Graph gallery. 2018. Accessed at: https://r-graph-gallery.com.

7. Rdocumentation. Glm fitting generalized linear models. Accessed at: https://www.rdocumentation.org/packages/stats/versions/3.6.2/topics/glm.

19 Survival Analysis

Survival Analysis

As opposed to traditional regressions discussed above, survival analyses take into consideration follow-up times instead of assuming every event has the same follow-up time; for example, if after being diagnosed with cancer, many patients are alive with that particular cancer, it makes a difference whether the follow-up occurred one week after surgery versus five years after surgery. Thus, the large difference with survival analysis is the consideration of what is called time-to-event data.

To perform survival analyses, we will need to download the following packages:

```
>Install.packages(survival)
>Install.packages(survminer)
>Install.packages(ggplot2)
```

We will additionally need to library the packages:

```
>library(survival)
>library(survminer)
>library(ggplot2)
```

Next, be sure to clean and import your data, as discussed in Chapter 18, and you are ready to perform the analysis. To perform this analysis, be sure to have in your line-by-line data the variables "survival," which should be the length of survival in months, and also a "vital" status with "1" signifying death and "0" signifying no death. You can also use this variable to signify recurrence and no recurrence with "1" and "0," respectively. This would assess progression-free survival.

Be sure to correctly key your death variable as "1" or recurrence as "1" instead of "0." If this is accidentally inverted, it will throw off all your results.

To make a comparison with the variable "race," we have the following formula to input:

```
>cox.cox <- coxph(Surv(Survival, Vitals) ~ Race)
```

With the return being similar to the following:

```
>summary(cox.cox)
Call: coxph(formula = Surv(Survival, Vitals) ~ Race)

  n= 126, number of events= 48

                coef   exp(coef)   se(coef)      z Pr(>|z|)
Race           0.7150   2.0442   0.2932 2.439   0.0147 *
---
Signif. codes:  0 '***' 0.001 '**' 0.01 '*' 0.05 '.' 0.1 ' ' 1

                exp(coef) exp(-coef) lower .95 upper .95
Race             2.044    0.4892    1.151    3.631

Concordance= 0.589  (se = 0.04 )
Likelihood ratio test= 5.91  on 1 df,   p=0.02
Wald test           = 5.95  on 1 df,   p=0.01
Score (logrank) test = 6.2  on 1 df,   p=0.01
```

As per these results, we can see that this race has a hazard ratio of 2.044 with a 95% confidence interval between 1.151 and 3.631. Instead of odds ratios, the survival analysis gives an assessment of a hazard where a value >1 indicates that the group has a worse survival rate than the control while having a hazard value <1 indicates that the group has a better survival rate than the control group. The p-value in this case is 0.0147.

As a single comparison, these are termed univariable Cox-regressions. For a multivariable Cox regression, we can perform this using the following more complex code string with many additional variables:

```
>cox.cox <- coxph(Surv(Survival, Vitals) ~ Race + Radiotherapy +
Sacrum + Male)
```

This results in the following output:

```
>summary(cox.cox)
Call:
coxph(formula = Surv(Osurv, Death) ~ Ages + Radiotherapy +
Sacrum + Male)

  n= 126, number of events= 26
```

	coef	exp(coef)	se(coef)	z	Pr(>|z|)
Race.	0.04958	1.05083.	0.01818	2.728	0.00637 **
Radiotherapy	0.30030	1.35027	0.41683	0.720	0.47126
Sacrum	1.10875	3.03057	0.74879	1.481	0.13868
Male	0.09478	1.09941.	0.43186	0.219	0.82629

```
---
Signif. codes:  0 '***' 0.001 '**' 0.01 '*' 0.05 '.' 0.1 ' ' 1
```

	exp(coef)	exp(-coef)	lower .95	upper .95
Race	1.051	0.9516	1.0141	1.089
Radiotherapy	1.350	0.7406	0.5965	3.057
Sacrum	3.031	0.3300	0.6985	13.149
Male	1.099	0.9096	0.4716	2.563

```
Concordance= 0.655  (se = 0.071 )
Likelihood ratio test= 10.64  on 4 df,   p=0.03
Wald test            = 9.78  on 4 df,   p=0.04
Score (logrank) test = 10.06  on 4 df,   p=0.04
```

Here, we can see that only "Race" is significant among the variables with a hazard ratio of 1.051 and a p-value of 0.00637.

Cox-Proportional Hazards Assumption

If performing a multivariable survival analysis model like this, it is important to consider the Cox-proportional hazards assumption. This assumption states that the ratio of hazards over the two tested cohorts remains constant over time. This can be tested via several different methods using Residuals.[1] Performing these diagnostics tests is supported by online resources[1] and is beyond the scope of this book; however, some journal reviewers may ask for this.

Finally, if we would like to fit a Kaplan–Meier plot for our manuscript, we can do this with the following script:

```
Fit <- survfit(Surv(Survival, Vitals) ~ Race, data=survival)
```

To create the plot (Fig. 19.1), we can input the following string:

```
>ggsurvplot(Fit, data=survival)
```

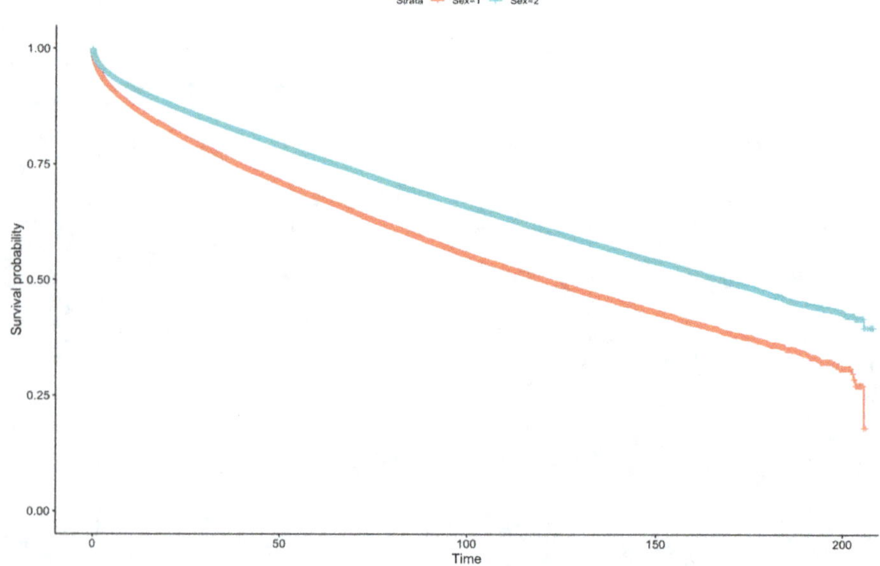

Fig. 19.1.   Overall Kaplan–Meier survival curve.

Additionally, if you would like to modify your charts, try the following code:

```
>ggsurvplot(Fit, data = NCDB_Tumor, size = 1, palette = c("#E7B800","#2E9FDF"), conf.int = TRUE, pval = TRUE, risk.table = TRUE, risk.table.col = "strata", legend.labs = c("Male", "Female"), risk.table.height = 0.25, ggtheme = theme_bw())
```

Which will output the following plot (Fig. 19.2):

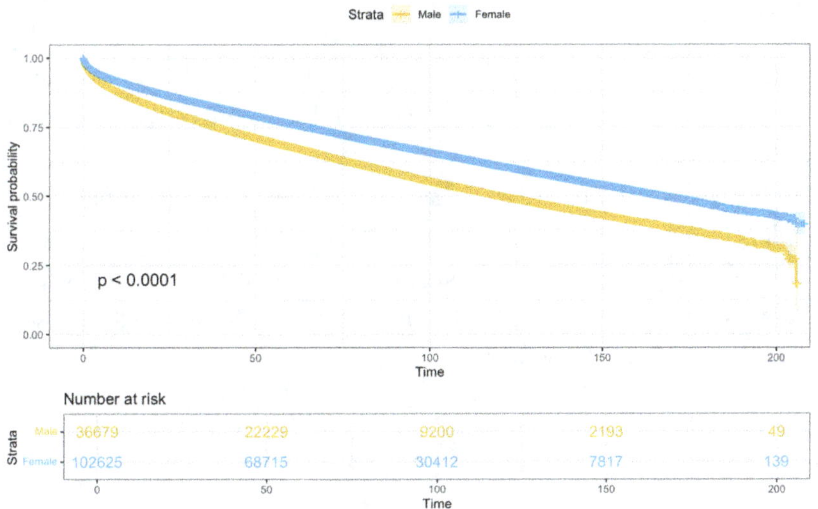

Fig. 19.2. Enhanced overall Kaplan–Meier survival curve.

In this figure, we can see a p-value in the bottom lift with a confidence interval associated with each cohort, as annotated by the blurred blue and yellow colors around the lines near the 200-month location. Additionally, a risk table is located at the bottom, which tells the reader how many exposed individuals are present at each time point of the analysis. Try to make your figure look like the figure above.

Further Figure Resources

For further ideas and code support with plots, check out The R Graph Gallery,[2] which includes great resources to find any figure that would be ideal for your particular manuscript. Additional helpful resources for performing survival analysis in RStudio can be found online at the Statistical Tools for High-Throughput Data Analysis website.[3]

References

1. Statistical Tools for High-Throughput Data Analysis. Cox model assumptions. Accessed at: https://www.sthda.com/english/wiki/cox-model-assumptions#google_vignette.
2. R Graph Gallery. The R Graph gallery. 2018. Accessed at: https://r-graph-gallery.com.
3. Statistical Tools for High-Throughput Data Analysis. Cox proportional-hazards model. Accessed at: https://www.sthda.com/english/wiki/cox-proportional-hazards-model.

20 Creating Predictive Calculators

Currently, a large and trending skill in clinical research is the use of machine learning and other different statistical algorithms to deliver precision medicine predictions. These often take the form of predictive calculators that can be employed with data and placed into peer-reviewed manuscripts.

In this chapter, we will discuss how to take your data and statistical models and create predictive calculators using the *Shiny* package in RStudio. We will discuss logistic/linear regression calculators.

Getting Ready

First, we will need to install the relevant packages that we will use for our script. To do this, we will input the following code:

```
>install.packages("shiny")
>install.packages("base64")
>install.packages("rsconnect")
>install.packages("shinythemes")
>install.packages("dplyr")
```

After doing this, all of the packages we need should be sufficiently installed in RStudio. Next, we will need to save the multivariable model that we would like to use in the calculator script. Let's start with the multivariable model and say we are attempting to create a multivariable model to detect invasion of the cavernous sinus in pituitary surgery. We create the following multivariable model using similar data principles, as discussed in Chapter 18:

```
>Invasion <- glm(formula = Invasion of cavernous sinus ~ Sex + Age + Somatotroph + Knosp + Dimension + Clinical Syndrome)
```

Since we have this model created saved as "Symptoms," we need to save this into a usable format to create our calculator. We will do this by inputting the following code:

```
>saveRDS(Invasion, "invasion.rds")
```

This will save our model as invasion.rds. Be sure to place your working directory on your desktop by clicking "Session" and "Working directory" at the top of RStudio. Once we have this saved, we can continue creating the calculator.

Writing the Calculator Script

Here, we will discuss the sections of the calculator code. This will include a summary of the sections followed by the actual code input into RStudio.

First, we need to library the packages that we have installed.

Second, this is where we will develop our fluid page, which is user-facing. We should add the title to this section and also have the option to make our available inputs as choices or continuous variables

At the end of this fluid section, we have a full text, which is typically labeled for your disclaimer of the calculator

This is where our previously saved model will be pulled into the calculator.

This must be saved in an .rds format.

This section of the script assigns your model variables to your user-facing fluid page.

This section of the script assigns your input and output.

```r
library(shiny)
library(base64)
library(rsconnect)
library(shinythemes)
library(dplyr)

ui <- fluidPage(


  titlePanel("Probability of Medial Wall Cavernous Sinus Invasion in
Pituitary Surgery"),


  sidebarLayout(
    sidebarPanel(
      selectInput("Sex", "Male or female?",
            choices=
              list(
                "Male"=1,
                "Female"=0),
              selected=0),
      sliderInput("Age", "Select age",
            min = 19.0, max = 89.0, value = 51.0),
      selectInput("Somatotroph",
            "Is the tumor a somatotroph?",
            choices=
              list(
                "Yes"=1,
                "No"=0),
              selected=0),
```

```r
selectInput("Knosp","Select Knosp grade",
      choices=
        list(
          "0"=0,
          "1"=1,
          "2"=2,
          "3A"=3,
          "3B"=4),
        selected=0),
  sliderInput("Dimension",
          "Select dimension (mm)",
          min = 3.00, max = 57.00, value = 20.0),
  selectInput("ClinicalSyndrome",
          "Is the tumor functional?",
          choices=
            list(
              "Yes"=1,
              "No"=0),
            selected=0)),

  mainPanel(
   tabsetPanel(type="tabs",
          tabPanel("Disclaimer",'The following calculator was cre-
ated on a retrospective cohort of 107 patients undergoing pituitary
tumor resection surgery at a single institution. This calculator has not
been externally validated. Please use with caution. Ultimately, the
treating neurosurgeon is responsible for optimizing patient care and
appropriate clinical decision making.


                   This model utilizes logistic regression
models to derive probability output. This calculator was rated with
the following c-statistic on a local dataset: Medial wall invasion 0.89.
All VIF parameters are measured <5 without colinearity. No local test-
ing dataset. No outer institutional testing dataset.'),
```

```
            tabPanel("Calculator Output",tableOutput("logit_table")))
      )
    )
)
server <- function(input, output) {

  wit <- readRDS("invasion.rds")

  finalmodel <- reactive({
   surv =
c((predict(wit,data.frame(Sex=as.integer(input$Sex),Age=as.integer
(input$Age),Somatotroph=as.integer(input$Somatotroph),
Knosp=as.integer(input$Knosp),Dimension=as.integer(input$
Dimension),ClinicalSyndrome=as.integer(input$ClinicalSyndrome)),
type="response")*100))
   surv[surv<=0]<-0
   surv[surv>=100]<-100

   data.frame(
     'Result' = c("Probability (%) of Cavernous Sinus Invasion"),
     'Output' = surv

   )})
  output$logit_table <- renderTable({
   finalmodel()
  })
}
shinyApp(ui=ui, server = server)
```

Deploying the Calculator

Once this is completed, we can click "Run App" at the top of the
script to test out our script. If it fails to work, check all periods,

commas, and variables. If something is not working, it is generally because the codes are not aligned properly, commas are not in appropriate spaces, or the variables are not spelled correctly. There are several additional online references for help with deploying shiny calculators.[2–5]

References

1. Shiny. Probability of medical wall cavernous sinus invasion in pituitary surgery. December 22, 2024. Accessed at: https://neurodx.shinyapps.io/Cavernousinvasion/.
2. Shiny. Gallery. December 22, 2024. Accessed at: https://shiny.posit.co/r/gallery/.
3. Shiny. Welcome to Shiny. Accessed at: https://shiny.posit.co/r/getstarted/shiny-basics/lesson1/.
4. Stats and R. How to publish a Shiny app? An example with shinyapps.io. May 29, 2020. Accessed at: https://statsandr.com/blog/how-to-publish-shiny-app-example-with-shinyapps-io/.
5. Medium. Shiny web applications for model deployment and visualization. Accessed at: https://medium.com/@msjntzkdt/unlocking-the-power-of-data-with-r-shiny-web-applications-for-model-deployment-and-visualisation-10fe0ff36281.

21 Meta-Analysis

The next type of analysis we will discuss is the meta-analysis.

To download the necessary packages, we will need to perform the following commands:

```
>install.packages("metafor")
```

And we will also need to library our package:

```
>library("metafor")
```

You will need to clean our data and make this into a usable format to run in RStudio. For the variables you want to use in your analysis, you would need to format your Excel spreadsheet appropriately.

The columns should be split into M1, SD1, and N1 to represent the mean value, standard deviation, and n-value for the first treatment you are measuring. Immediately next to these columns should be M2, SD2, and N2 for the mean value, standard deviation, and n-value for your comparative treatment, respectively. Each row should have different values found in each study (Fig. 21.1).

You additionally need to import and attach our data "Search_ Data" using the flow described in Chapter 18:

G1		A	B	C	D	E	F
1		M1	SD1	N1	M2	SD2	N2
2							
3							
4							
5							
6							

Fig. 21.1.   Microsoft Excel formatting for meta-analysis in RStudio.

In the first part of the analysis, we will calculate the effect sizes and their variance. You can do this with the following string:

```
>model <- escalc(measure="SMD", m1i=M1 sd1i=SD1, n1i=N1,
m2i=M2, sd2i=SD2, n2i=N2, data=Search_Data, append = TRUE)
```

Let's say we would like to compare mean averages among studies, otherwise known as a standardized mean difference of the studies. We can do that by inputting the following code for performing a random-effects meta-analysis:

```
>heterotest <- rma(yi, vi, data=Search_Data)
```

Next, we will call for a summary of the random effects model:

```
>summary(heterotest)
```

Next, after calling a summary, it will give you an output that looks like this:

```
Random-Effects Model (k = 7; tau^2 estimator: REML)

 logLik deviance    AIC    BIC    AICc
-4.9350   9.8700  13.8700  13.4535  17.8700

tau^2 (estimated amount of total heterogeneity): 0.2462 (SE = 0.1745)
tau (square root of estimated tau^2 value): 0.4962
```

```
I^2 (total heterogeneity / total variability): 85.63%
H^2 (total variability / sampling variability): 6.96

Test for Heterogeneity:
Q(df = 6) = 38.1639, p-val < .0001

Model Results:

estimate    se    zval   pval   ci.lb   ci.ub
 -0.5708  0.2082  -2.7419  0.0061  -0.9788  -0.1628  **

---
Signif. codes:  0 '***' 0.001 '**' 0.01 '*' 0.05 '.' 0.1 ' ' 1
```

This is where we have our p-value and estimate with confidence intervals. Notice that our I^2 value is =85.63%, which represents heterogenous data. If the I^2 was <50%, we could consider the use of a fixed-effects model for meta-analysis.

Let's say we wanted to perform a meta-analysis but would like to use a fixed-effects model. This would be done with the following string where method = "FE" is inserted:

```
>heterotest <- rma(yi, vi, data=Search_Data, method = "FE")
```

Let's say we wanted to make a forest plot with our created meta-analysis model information:

```
>forest(model, xlab = "Mean difference", slab = c("Hiyama et al,
2022", "Penalosa et al, 2021", "Barone et al, 2021", "Kawabata et al,
2022", "Yagi et al, 2021", "Noh et al, 2020 (Derivation)", "Noh et al,
2020 (Validation)"), showweights = TRUE, pch = 17, ilab = cbind
(Search_Data$n1i, Search_Data$m1i,Search_Data$sd1i, Search_
Data$n2i, Search_Data$m2i, Search_Data$sd2i), ilab.xpos = c(-3.1,
-2.7,-2.1,-1.6,-1.1,-0.7))
```

Additionally, a funnel plot to test for publication bias can be assessed using the following formula as well:

```
>funnel(heterotest, main="Standard Error")
>funnel(heterotest I, yaxis="vi", main="Sampling Variance")
>funnel(heterotest, yaxis="seinv", main="Inverse Standard Error")
>funnel(heterotest, yaxis="vinv", main="Inverse Sampling Variance")
```

You can even run a test for asymmetry of your funnel plots:

```
>regtest(heterotest)
```

Additional references for using RStudio to complete meta-analyses can be found online.[1-6]

References

1. Rdocumentation. escalc: Calculating effect sizes and outcome measures. Accessed at: https://www.rdocumentation.org/packages/metafor/versions/3.8-1/topics/escalc.
2. The Comprehensive R Archive Network. Metafor: Meta-analysis package for R. March 28, 2024. Accessed at: https://cran.r-project.org/web/packages/metafor/metafor.pdf.
3. Rdocumentation. Metafor-package: Metafor: A meta-analysis package for R. Accessed at: https://www.rdocumentation.org/packages/metafor/versions/0.5-3/topics/metafor-package.
4. The metafor package: A meta-analysis package for R. Analysis examples. 2024. Accessed at: https://www.metafor-project.org/doku.php/analyses.
5. Viechtbauer W. Conducting meta-analyses in R with the metafor package. *Journal of Statistical Software*. 2010; **36**. Accessed at: https://cran.r-project.org/web/packages/metafor/vignettes/metafor.pdf.
6. RPubs by RStudio. Tutorial: Running meta-analysis in R using the metafor package. 2013. Accessed at: https://rpubs.com/jokel/10913.

Part V
Achieving the End Goal

22 Basics of Writing a Manuscript

Once you have completed the data analysis, the next step will be to write the manuscript. Writing a manuscript is equally important as performing the actual data analysis because if a paper is difficult to read and interpret, this will significantly limit the way individuals view your results. Plenty of novel studies have been performed with great significance in the literature that, when published, were poorly written. As a result, these studies did not get published in good journals and were not readily assessed by the scientific community due to poor writing.

In this chapter, we will discuss the basics of writing a manuscript and how to make your hypothesis and the findings of your study easy for the reader to grasp.

Overall Formatting

To format a manuscript to be submission-ready, most manuscript documents should be submitted as Microsoft Word files (see Appendix 2). It is best to label each page with page numbers in the bottom right corner of the document. Additionally, line numbers can be placed throughout the manuscript. Line spacing should also be double-spaced.

It is important to note that these are basic guidelines and may be subject to change, depending on which journal you are submitting. Most writers begin with a basic Word document and then modify this document until submission to a journal, according to journal guidelines. If the paper is rejected, they will still have the basic document and can modify it again for another journal. Journal guidelines are usually displayed on websites under "Author guidelines."

Most journal websites will specifically give you the maximum word count, maximum table, maximum figure count, and reference styles for their journals. It is imperative to follow these instructions carefully, as incorrect formatting can reduce your overall manuscript score and lead to a rejection when the paper could have initially been accepted.

Parts of the Manuscript

After formatting your initial document, you can begin writing — it is paramount that the manuscript be kept clean, concise, and easy to read. When writing, imagine your reader being a busy healthcare professional who only has a small amount of time. If you are fortunate that the busy healthcare professional reads past the abstract, your text should be as clean and concise as possible for the reader.

Title Page

The title page is the first page of your manuscript document. It begins with a title at the very top of the page, with the authorship order immediately below the title. The authors should be spelled with their first name, middle initial, and last name, along with their highest degrees. Superscripts will denote author affiliation and affiliation location. The authorship order is additionally important. The person performing the study would be considered the first author, with the most senior author being in the very last spot. The middle of the authorship order generally goes from the most junior to senior author. Be very clear to all authors about what the authorship order will be and, if possible, be very clear before even beginning the study.

Finally, the lower portion of the title page should be the corresponding author, which is generally the senior author of the manuscript. In this location, you will list the corresponding author's full name, title, affiliation, email address, and mailing address. It is also worth mentioning that many journals allow for pre-publication corresponding authors and post-publication corresponding authors. This essentially lets a more junior person complete the submission process but allows the principal investigator to be the point of contact for individuals reading the study once it is actually in circulation with the peer-reviewed journal.

> Be very clear on who will be the corresponding author on your manuscripts. Some principal investigators prefer junior individuals to be the corresponding authors, and some prefer the principal investigator to be the corresponding author.

Abstract

After the title page, the abstract is essentially a synopsis of every aspect of the paper. Case reports and literature reviews will typically have unstructured abstracts, while every other type will be split into introduction, methods, results, and conclusions. Many individuals will complete the abstract as the last step of the manuscript submission process since it is just an overview of the entire manuscript. Overall, it is good practice to have the results section of the abstract be the largest portion. Many journals limit the abstract to 250 to 300 words.

Keywords

After the abstract, the manuscript typically will list 5–7 keywords, each separated by semicolons. These will be used by PubMed for indexing purposes and can drastically affect your manuscript being identified in a search. Be sure to use smart keywords for your study that accurately describe your article.

Introduction

The first writing section of the manuscript is the introduction. Here, the author introduces the problem and narrows it down to the hypothesis of the study being tested. The introduction can be thought of very broadly as an inverted triangle. In your first paragraph, you want to start by explaining your large problem or disease you are targeting. How problematic are the issues? How many people does it affect worldwide? Is it a very debilitating disease? Overall, you are trying to make a case to the journal reviewers as to why they should accept your article. Therefore, from the beginning, you should explain how big of a problem the issue you are studying is in the world. In the next paragraph, you should explain what is causing this big problem to happen. What is leading to this trouble? As you can see, we are trying to narrow down our final study hypothesis. Lastly, in the third paragraph, you should specifically state in a single clear and concise sentence the primary objective of your study. Additionally, if you have any secondary objectives, it is appropriate to list them in the final paragraph.

With this three-paragraph flow to your introduction, you keep your introduction quick and concise, and you effectively explain your case to the reviewers why what you are studying is a big problem and how your study addresses that problem. It is essential to keep your introduction concise and coherent, as this is the readers'

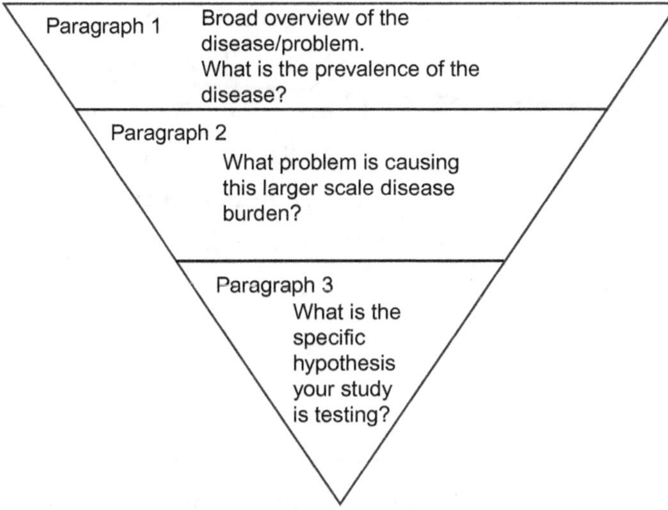

Fig. 22.1.   Writing the introduction to the article.

first interaction with your writing. Have you ever read a study with such a lengthy introduction that you became so bored you gave up reading the entire study altogether? It happens. Medical professionals are busy people so keep your introduction clear and concise with this three-paragraph format (Fig. 22.1).

Methods

After your introduction, the next section will be on your methods. This will significantly vary depending on the type of manuscript you are developing. It is best to split your methods section by subheadings. One of your first subheadings should be your recruitment or search strategy. This will include any required comment on IRB approval or exemption. It will additionally explain information on any databases you may have used to retrieve patient information. This includes database search codes and search criteria. Strict inclusion and exclusion criteria should be included. Next, there should be a section on statistical analysis, specifically describing which tests were used for what comparisons. Additionally, it should explain all the statistical software that was used and with the appropriate version and updates. Additionally, any packages used should be disclosed. Finally, a section on bias or quality should be included. This includes detecting publication bias in meta-analyses or performing the Newcastle-Ottawa[1] grading system for quality scoring.

Results

This is one of the most important sections of your manuscript. Here, you will report all your results. Generally speaking, your results will have the following format:

- Number of patients included in each cohort
- Baseline comparisons of the two included cohorts (Are the intervention groups and non-intervention groups similar in baseline demographics and comorbidities?)
- Initial bivariable comparisons of the treatment and control group (Directly testing the hypothesis)
- Multivariable comparison of the treatment and control group (Testing the hypothesis while controlling for other potential confounders).

As you can see from these points, the results section is listed from the most basic comparisons to the adjusted and more advanced modeling. Tables and figures should be used extensively in this section to make the results section easier to read. Make the results section easy to read, such that if a medical professional reads the results only, it is easily understandable. Conciseness is key.

Discussion

In the Discussion section, your goal is to take your newly found data and incorporate these new findings into existing literature. There are several methods to writing this section, and generally, there is no universal way to do so. One good method is to have your first paragraph be an overview of your study's significant findings. What important findings did you have in 3–5 sentences? After this initial paragraph, many people will take one finding per paragraph and compare it with the current literature. Therefore, if you think you have four significant findings, you should have four paragraphs in the discussion after the initial summary paragraph. You should discuss any values that were found to be statistically significant in your study. All discussion sections should include a final subsection entitled "Limitations." Every study should have limitations explicitly annotated in this section. No study is without limitations; do not keep this section light because you think your paper will stand a better chance of being accepted to better journals. It is actually the reverse — the more limitations you point out, the more robust your piece of work actually is to the scientific community. Another potential subsection you can include is "Future research," which will suggest the next step(s) to the readers for future investigations. These could be investigations you are doing yourself or some ideas that other investigators can tackle.

Conclusions

Your conclusion should include 2–3 sentences incorporating your most novel finding, how it fits into the current literature, and what is to be performed next in this area. If you wanted the readers to remember 2–3 sentences, what would they be? When writing this section, it can be helpful to think: if a busy individual were only able to review the conclusion, what would I want this person to know?

References

References will be placed after the Conclusion section of the manuscript. It is important to adhere to the author guidelines for this section. Most journals will directly list how many references are allowed and even provide examples of citations at the end of the manuscript. Text citations also vary and can range from superscripts to brackets within the text. This section is important — many journals will return your work if there are no appropriate reference sections or just reject your manuscript outright.

Figure Legend

After your Reference section, most journals would like your figure legends to be included inside the manuscript document. You can list them here. Be sure to look up the author guidelines for formatting your figure legends.

Tables

Most tables will be submitted in separate Word documents. Overall, general requirements for tables can vary but are also explicitly annotated on any journal's author guidelines. Abbreviations and footnotes should be added at the bottom of the table. Tables should be typed using the Arial font for easy readability and are generally submitted in a separate Microsoft Word document.

Figures

Figures are generally submitted as completely separate and isolated files. They should be shared in high-resolution Tagged Image File Format (TIFF) or PDFs. These can easily be produced using Microsoft Powerpoint or Apple Keynote and exported into these file types. This is a very convenient way to produce figures, as you can add text boxes, shapes, and other objects onto your figures. Once done, click "File" and export them to either a TIFF or PDF file format. Once exported, most journals require a minimum of 300 DPI for color figures and 600 DPI for black-and-white images. This can be tricky. On a MacBook, you can adjust the sizing using the program Preview. However, if you do not have a program to perform this on your computer, there are many online size converters that are available. Journals usually will not hold this requirement for you until after your manuscript is accepted. However, most journals do have some pre-acceptance requirements for figures, which vary widely from journal to journal. Most journals will want you to crop out erroneous figure borders and label the figures according to journal criteria.

Cover Letters

Finally, once everything is ready for submission, your manuscript should be accompanied by a cover letter. This is essentially a letter on top of your manuscript that states the novel findings of the manuscript and how these fit into the submitted journal's readership. This cover letter should be placed on an institutional letterhead from the principal investigator and be signed by the principal investigator.

Plagiarism Check

Every investigator has different routines for detecting internal plagiarism. One of the best ways to make sure what you submit is not plagiarized is to run the entire paper through an online plagiarism tracker before submission. These can easily be found on websites, such as the Chegg.com Writing Center[2] or Grammarly.com.[3] Failure to detect plagiarism can lead to significant consequences.

Most journals screen every submitted manuscript using the iThenticate software.[4] This software is able to detect plagiarism from a significant amount of resources and, more recently, is also able to identify AI-produced material.[4] If you submit a manuscript with a significant amount of plagiarized material, this is a serious issue, and, at a minimum, your article will be immediately rejected. More adverse consequences can include referral to your institutional professionalism committee for evaluation and other institutional-related punishments.

This is a very difficult concept because we may not know who has helped write our manuscripts in many cases. Oftentimes, more junior students assist in writing. Additionally, students from other institutions may also have been involved in the preparation. Other individuals, when gathering information, may not even know if they are plagiarizing from other sources. To fight this ambiguity, one of the best ways is to get into the habit of screening every manuscript you have using an online plagiarism tracker before submiting it. Most academic journals have a 15% threshold for similarity, while fiction-related writing can be lower at around 10%.[5] It is best to have the similarity percentage as close to 0% as possible. It is just not worth the risk. Submitting one significantly plagiarized paper is enough to make getting >20% accepted not worth it. Get into the habit of submitting every manuscript through a validated plagiarism tracker.

Plagiarism in manuscripts is a significant issue once it is submitted to a journal. Be sure to run your manuscript through a plagiarism detector before submission!

Once all these items are complete, congratulations! You are now ready to submit your manuscript to a journal!

References

1. OHRI. Newcastle-Ottawa Quality Assessment Scale case control studies. 2000. Accessed at: https://www.ohri.ca/programs/clinical_epidemiology/nosgen.pdf.

2. Chegg. Plagiarism. 2024. Accessed at: https://www.chegg.com/writing/features/plagiarism-checker?c_id=sem&utm_source=google&utm_medium=cpc&utm_campaign=cw--head_terms_US_ai_catchall_broad&utm_content=ai+plagiarism+checker&gad_source=1&gbraid=0AAAAADuui-Z7Yomkb7LJv-HdvF0JPXIo7R&gclid=CjwKCAiAmrS7BhBJEiwAei59i7efgH4zMJOYlfCzlr46b9linX0CgN5fpG4CMOd09IGX5NG7vJGTJhoCFo-8QAvD_BwE&gclsrc=aw.ds.

3. Grammarly. Plagiarism checker. 2024. Accessed at: https://www.grammarly.com/plagiarism-checker.

4. iThenticate. Publish with confiedence. 2024. Accessed at: https://www.ithenticate.com.

5. Antonio J, Garib A. Editor's message: Sufficient details in a manuscript, originality, and similarity score. 2022. *Journal of Microwave Power and Electromagnetic Energy*. **56**: 69–70. Accessed at: https://www.tandfonline.com/doi/full/10.1080/08327823.2022.2071810.

Chapter 23 Selecting and Submitting to Journals

Now that you have completed your writing portion, congratulations! You are now ready to submit your work for publication.

Originally, it was intended that investigators would first present their idea to a conference, obtain feedback, and then begin a full manuscript. We will discuss that process here.

Selecting Conferences for Presentations

First, it would be best to submit your work to a conference. Overall, your work should only be submitted to one national conference and possibly one local conference. Find a national conference in your field; most medical specialties will have some form of national body organization that has an annual meeting to include research presentations. The reasons for submitting to these conferences are two-fold: to be able to present your research in front of national leaders in your field, and this is great for networking purposes as you can meet leaders and innovators across the nation. It is beneficial to attend these conferences even if you are not presenting, if not just solely for this purpose. National conferences are typically considered the gold standard presentations for your work.

Once submitted, most conferences will have three main types of presentations that you will be accorded. The types of presentations can vary. However, they are generally in some form of electronic poster, print poster, short oral presentation, or full presentation. Electronic posters are displayed on a revolving screen at the conference and are the least desired, generally speaking. A print poster ensures your poster is up during the entire conference for people to view. However, there will be a set timeframe (usually a couple of hours) where individuals can stand next to their poster and do a two-minute presentation where conference attendees can ask questions. Sometimes, during this process, there is also a poster competition where your two-minute speech is rated against your peers. The next two types of presentations are oral presentations, where you deliver a podium talk to conference attendees. A short presentation is generally <15 minutes in length in a small room of people interested in that subspecialty. However, the full oral presentation, or plenary presentation, can last up to 30 minutes and may involve the entire conference at a general meeting of the convention. Obviously, the latter option is the most desired, and it is typically reserved for very novel and significant developments. Overall, the goal at this stage is to obtain feedback for your study and incorporate it into your future full manuscript.

Of note, there are additional conferences that you can attend in the form of local conferences, where you can obtain feedback from local peers but may not necessarily take the place of a national conference. Examples of this could include local medical school research days and local medical specialty society group organizations. Another conference you may have the opportunity to present would be at an international or global medical society. It is generally considered that national figures do not attend these and thus are adjunctive conferences mainly related to global reach projects. Therefore, for studies, national conferences are usually the best choices for your work.

Selecting Journals for Submission

When considering medical journals, there are two significant types of journals you must consider: basic science journals and clinical journals. Depending on what kind of study you have, this will significantly narrow down your journal selection process. Journals like *Science* and *Nature* are good examples of basic science journals while *JAMA* and *Lancet* typically publish more clinical articles. You would not want to submit your clinical articles to journals that only publish basic science research. Given that this book was written to assist in clinical research only, we will place particular emphasis on these types of journals.

Subscription versus Open Access Journals

Another key differentiator in journals that we will discuss is subscription-based journals versus open access journals. Most clinical journals are subscription-based journals. The business model of these journals consists of authors submitting their research work to the journal for publication at no price to whoever is submitting the work. As a result, the price is borne by the readers of the articles in the form of a journal subscription. This is considered the most traditional way of having your manuscript accepted to a journal. One downside of this model is that readers who do not have the ability to pay to read the articles in the journal will be unable to view the material. Thus, subscription publications may have less visibility to the scientific community when compared to open access material.

The next type of model is termed "open access journals." This occurs when the authors submit their work to a journal and, if accepted, pay the cost to publish the articles so that readers can view the work for free. Open access fees can typically range from $2,000 to $4,000 per publication and can vary based on the journal and type of publication. Most open access journals are easier to publish your work in because you have to pay an article-processing fee first. Some journals have the option to publish either by subscription or by open access. Check with your institutional library as well since many institutions have publication agreements with certain journals that allow for a complete publication fee waiver.

> Be very sure that you have the funds to publish an open access manuscript with the associated article processing fees. If you do not have the money to pay for an open access publication, but yet the work is accepted, you have essentially lost a lot of time in this submission process when you could have been submitting to a subscription journal.

The Journal Submission Flowthrough

It is best to consider your journal selection process as a tiered approach (Fig. 23.1). Your first journals where you initially submit will be reach journals (chances of minimal acceptances). Even though it can be a hassle to submit to these journals, it is important, as the key to getting accepted to large impact factor journals is multiple submissions. Many large impact factor journals, such as *JAMA* and *Lancet*, have acceptance rates of around 5–10%.[1,2] Therefore, for every ten articles you submit, you would do well to get one acceptance. However, if you are looking for quick acceptances, this would be the step to bypass. A good thing about these types of journals is that they often have a quick and robust editor desk rejection capability, so you don't get held up for multiple

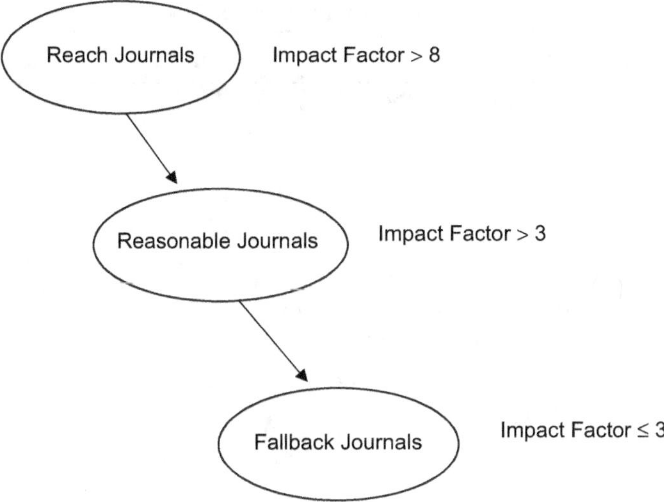

Fig. 23.1.   Flow of journal submissions.

months sending to these journals with very low rates of acceptances; these often let you know within a week of a decision.

It is important to consider when submitting your manuscript that you are not allowed to submit your work to multiple journals at the same time. For example, you should not submit your work to a top-tier journal, a middle-tier journal, and a lower tier simultaneously. This is because submitting to multiple journals at the same time is a waste of reviewers' time, which is generally viewed as a valuable commodity to the journals and their editorial staff. Additionally, no work should be published twice in two different journals. All previous conference presentations should also be annotated with a journal submission on the cover letter or editorial submission system.

When selecting journals for submission, it is helpful to use the impact factor system explained in Chapter 2. As of the publication of this book, the following is a list of top medical journals for medical research (Table 23.1).

Table 23.1.   List of Journal h5-Indexes[3]

Rating	Publication	h5-index	h5-median
1	*The New England Journal of Medicine*	434	897
2	*The Lancet*	368	678
3	*JAMA*	298	498
4	*Nature Medicine*	274	474
5	*Proceedings of the National Academy of Sciences*	267	405
6	*International Journal of Molecular Sciences*	244	346
7	*PLOS ONE*	225	322
8	*BMJ*	224	388
9	*JAMA Network Open*	177	267
10	*Cell Metabolism*	160	240

Obviously, not every manuscript will get accepted to one of these top-tier journals. However, it would be a nice thing to have. Some investigators strive their entire careers to be accepted at such a journal. Luckily, many other top-tier journals employ a quick editorial desk rejection system where the first decision on your manuscript will be reached in less than a week. Therefore, most of the time required is dedicated largely to formatting the manuscript for submission and actually submitting the manuscript. If your manuscript is rejected by one of these journals, they may give you the option to automatically transfer your manuscript to an open access journal.

If your manuscript is rejected by one of the top-tier journals, the next journal to submit to would be in the moderate impact range. To do this, look online for journals in your field that have an impact factor of around 8 to 3. These would be considered moderate impact factor journals that a reasonably carried out and developed study should obtain acceptance. Submitting to these journals will typically consist of a review period of 2–3 months. If this were rejected, it would be reasonable to submit your work to a lower-tier journal that has less than an impact factor of 3 for your particular field of interest. At this point, if it is rejected from a low-tier journal, it is best to submit it to multiple low-tier journals. Most clinical manuscripts will get accepted in the middle- to low-tier journal range.

If you are still not able to secure an acceptance at any of the low-tier journals and you feel that you have adequately submitted your work to almost all the relevant journals in your field, there are other options. Some journals take pride in "transparent publishing," where they report accepting almost all manuscripts that are proofread, are performed with ethics, and have clear analysis. These journals take pride in accepting every manuscript to eliminate the wall that can sometimes be made by journals in a particular field, barring certain ideas from publication. A couple of these journals are *Cureus*[4] and *Heliyon*.[5] Do note that it will cost authors to publish in these journals. These journals are also PubMed-indexed and are considered peer-reviewed.

Non-Peer Reviewed Publications

Another option is publishing your work to a pre-print server. These server sites include the ability to publish a manuscript online and are intended to publish your work while it is in the submission process. However, if you are unable to obtain true admission, you can also just be published here as well. Examples of routinely used pre-print servers would include arXiv[6] and bioRxiv.[7] Work in pre-print journals has become exceedingly common (Fig. 23.2).

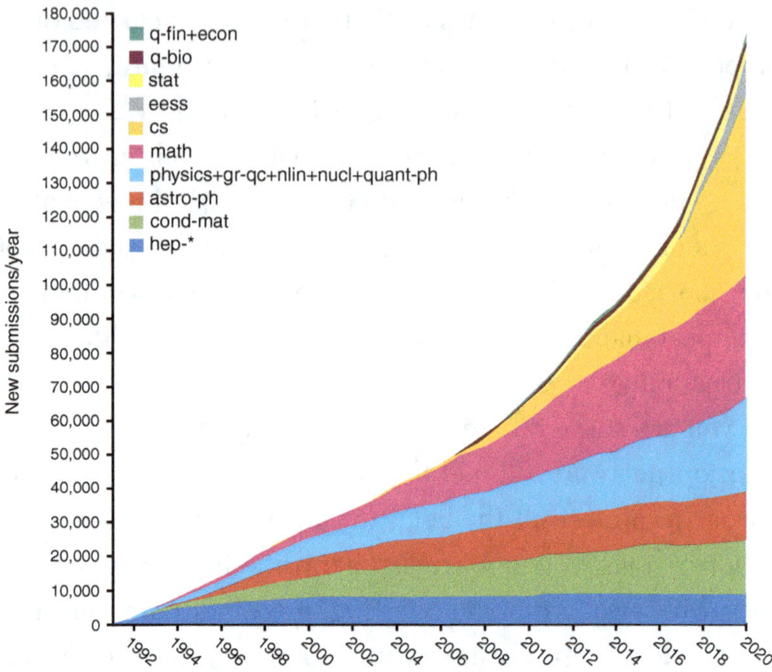

Fig. 23.2.   ArXiv's yearly submission rate growth over 30 years since its beginning.[8]

These were originally designed to allow scientists to publicly share their work online before submission and acceptance to academic journals. This allows scientists to publicly disseminate their results and obtain feedback before submission. Once accepted for publication in a full journal, these pre-prints can be removed. Some pre-print servers, such as arXiv, also offer the option to be indexed on PubMed. Typically, academic journals allow for pre-print journals.

Predatory Journals: A Word of Caution

When searching for a home for your manuscript, there are certain criteria you should always search for. First and foremost, be absolutely sure that your journal is indexed in PubMed. There are really only very few reasons and special circumstances why you would publish in a non-PubMed indexed journal; however, that is beyond the scope of this book. Additionally, this should only really be done with more experienced investigators. To check this, journals typically have a list of indexed sources on their "About me" page. Additionally, you can also always run a PubMed search and make sure the journal is indexed by finding other manuscripts from that journal on PubMed.

Once you are sure that a journal is included on PubMed, make sure your journal is not on Beall's List of predatory journals.[9] Jeffrey Beall was an American librarian who published a list of "predatory" journals in 2011. These journals solicit requests for manuscripts with quick and easy publication in return for an open-access fee. It was eventually discovered that these journals often employ no peer-review process (or their peer-review processes are so easy that they have no scientific merit). Essentially, the journals will publish any manuscript as long as the author pays a fee. This may be an easy route at first; however, most experienced researchers know which are the predatory journals in their field, and if you were to publish in these journals, it would not look very advantageous. Additionally, once the article is published, it is impossible to erase. The article will continue to be on PubMed and be discovered in plagiarism databases. Make all attempts to avoid predatory journals.

Another word of caution is to avoid all email solicitations for "free article publications" and "article requests." These entities will often take your manuscript and publish it on their website, which has no scientific merit. Thus, it also cannot be taken down and will show up on any future plagiarism scans. Thus, if your work ever shows up on one of these predatory websites, most reasonable academic journals will no longer consider publishing this work.

References

1. JAMA Netowork. For authors. Accessed at: https://jamanetwork.com/journals/jama/pages/for-authors#:~:text=Editorial%20Information.,than%205%2C000%20research%20manuscripts%20received.

2. Lancet. Information for authors. December, 2024. Accessed at: https://www.thelancet.com/pb-assets/Lancet/authors/tl-info-for-authors-1690986041530.pdf.

3. Google Scholar. Top publications. 2024. Accessed at: https://scholar.google.com/citations?view_op=top_venues&hl=en&vq=med_medgeneral.

4. Cureus. Main webpage. 2024. Accessed at: https://www.cureus.com.

5. Heliyon: Cell Press. Main webpage. 2024. Accessed at: https://www.cell.com/heliyon/home.

6. arXiv. Main webpage. 2024. Accessed at: https://arxiv.org.

7. bioXiv. Main webpage. 2024. Accessed at https://www.biorxiv.org.

8. Paul Ginsparg. August 4, 2021. Accessed at: https://upload.wikimedia.org/wikipedia/commons/0/0d/ArXiv%27s_yearly_submission_rate_plot.jpg.

9. Beall's List. Beall's list of potential predatory journals and publishers. December 8, 2021. Accessed at: https://beallslist.net/.

24 The Journal Review Process and Responding to Revisions

Once you have found and submitted your work to the appropriate journal, congratulations. Now, it is out of your hands! For an overview of the journal review process, it operates in the following manner. First, the journal is a private and for-profit entity. It employs an editor-in-chief, who is in charge of publication and the editorial process. Additionally, many journals will have a deputy editor and associate editors. The types of editors can significantly change with the type of journal, the journal size, and the field of the journal.

When you submit to a journal, the manuscript is formally submitted to the editor-in-chief (hence, that's why the cover letter is to be addressed to this person). Here, it will initially undergo an administrative review that will assess for correct manuscript formatting in accordance with the author guidelines of that journal. From there, the editor-in-chief will route the manuscript to a more junior editor. This more junior editor may be an editor overseeing a specific focus of the journal. From there, if the editors find the manuscript worthy of peer review, they will send the manuscript for peer review.

The peer reviewers vary widely across different journals. Some journals are very prestigious, so reviewing for those types of journals is viewed as a significant honor, and the reviewers are generally esteemed individuals in the field. Other smaller journals solicit their reviews from more casual reviewers who are solicited to perform peer reviews. Peer reviewers for each manuscript are journal and editor-dependent, and you can expect to encounter 1–4 peer reviewers during the journal's peer-review process.

During the peer-review process, the reviewers will annotate what they think your strengths are with the manuscript and where you can improve. Confidentially to the editor, they will also suggest whether the editor should reject or accept your manuscript. Eventually, all of these comments are forwarded to the author for constructive feedback, along with possible comments from an editor.

It is very important to understand that most of getting an article accepted is very random with multiple factors. For example, some editors may deliver a more positive response to manuscripts more consistently than other editors. Some peer reviewers may also be more positive than other peer reviewers. The journal may have had a very recent study published last month. There is really a good portion of randomness found in these journals with respect to getting an article accepted. It is important to view this process from strength and consider all feedback from reviewers as knowledge taken to improve your manuscript. Do not take it personally!

Additionally, there is also ambiguity over whether the author's identity will lead to more acceptances in many journals. It is currently very ambiguous whether authors of the manuscript play a role in the acceptance process. Many journals suggest a "blind review" process. However, it is typically not specified at which point the review process becomes blind. Do the peer reviewers know the names of the authors? Do the section editors? Does the editor-in-charge? It is largely left ambiguous in most journals.

Additionally, some fields and subfields in medicine are so small that it is almost impossible to make the reviewers completely blind to authorship with some studies. If a study comes across a journal with a certain treatment or technique, and there is only one medical faculty at one institution performing this procedure, it is difficult to blind this particular type of work.

Receiving the Response

Once fully submitted, there are five main types of responses that you will see with journals:

- **Editor desk rejection**
  Used by larger journals. Once submitted, the paper will be reviewed by a journal editor. The editor finds the manuscript either out of the scope of the journal or not having enough merit to be considered for peer review. This typically manifests as a rejection only a few days after submission. This is helpful for authors submitting to journals with low acceptance rates because it does not result in the author submitting their work to a journal with a 10% acceptance rate after four months of waiting for a response.
- **Rejection after peer-review**
  This occurs when the author submits a manuscript to a journal, and the editors of the journal believe it has the merit for peer review. It is sent to the peer reviewers but is rejected outright with no chance of revision after peer review.
- **Major revision**
  This occurs once a manuscript has made it to peer review and the peer reviewers believe it is acceptable for publication in the journal, but significant changes are needed before publication.

This typically will be in the format of either significantly revising written text, re-selecting patients, or re-performing some aspects of data analysis. Generally speaking, if you receive an update stating that your manuscript needs major revision, it generally will end up being accepted as long as the necessary changes are made. For accepted papers, this is the most likely decision you will initially receive.

- **Minor revision**

  This occurs once a manuscript has made it to peer review and the peer reviewers believe it is acceptable for publication in the journal but slight modifications are needed. This will typically come in the form of the reviewers requesting you to change a few sentences of the writing or manipulate tables and figures. If you receive this response, you will most likely be accepted once the necessary revisions are made.

- **Acceptance without revision**

  This occurs when the peer-reviewers deem your article acceptable without any modifications. Otherwise known as accepted "as is," this is a very rare occurrence.

Receiving a Rejection

After receiving a rejection, it is important to take the feedback for the journal and incorporate it as best as you can in the manuscript.

First, what was the reason? Was the manuscript too far out of the scope for that particular journal? If so, this could mean your journal search strategy needs fine-tuning. Return to Chapter 23 for the journal selection process. For first-time submitters, it is important to read the scope of the journal you are submitting to.

If it was within the scope of the journal but the Editor's Desk rejected the manuscript, they would usually leave comments. Attempt to address these comments and submit your manuscript elsewhere. In most cases of a desk reject, there is no option to submit to that journal a second time. If you obtained a desk reject with no comments, just quickly submit it elsewhere. Desk rejection without any comments typically is done by very high-impact factor journals with significantly low acceptance rates.

Do not get discouraged by rejections! It is typical for manuscripts to be rejected ~3–4 times before eventually gaining acceptance.

Receiving a Revision

Congratulations! If you have received an update that your manuscript requires major or minor revision, your likelihood of acceptance is high.

For major revisions, this usually means the reviewers feel your article has merit but needs substantial revision. Perform the edits that the reviewers are suggesting and change the text with the "Track Changes" in Microsoft Word. Additionally, answer all critiques made by the reviewers on a reviewer response document. Such an example can be found in Appendix 3. It is best to directly answer the reviewers for each point while also listing line-by-line responses stating what was added to the manuscript. Therefore, at the end of this process, you should have addressed all of your reviewers' responses. Making each part of the response color-coded for easier reading by the editors and peer-reviewers is also helpful. If all of the reviewers feel like you have addressed their comments, you likely will get accepted. If they believe that it needs an additional revision, they may return the manuscript to you with a second major revision or a subsequent minor revision to complete. Minor revisions are very similar to how you respond to the reviewers.

> Be sure to address all reviewer comments directly! Rejections at the revision stage usually occur when writers fail to directly address one or multiple reviewer comments.

When responding to the reviewers, keep the responses cordial, professional, and constructive. Do not argue with reviewers or state you will not make those changes. If they request something that you are not able to perform, list this in the limitations section. Generally speaking, you do not want to argue with reviewers unless you are willing to submit it to another journal entirely, and at the beginning of your career, there really is no need to argue with reviewers in this stage of the process.

Once you have completed all your reviewers' responses and have created a reviewer response document, return your submission to the journal, where the editors will oversee whether you addressed the reviewers' concerns adequately (or not). In some cases, they may send the revision back for re-review as well. If addressed well, they will accept your paper. Congratulations!

After Acceptance

Once accepted, the editor will send you a formal acceptance email. For your CV purposes, the article is listed as "Accepted" or "In press" until full publication of the article. From here, you will wait for the journal production team to send you a proof of the article in the final PDF format as to how it will appear in the journal. This is your opportunity to make any final changes. At a minimum, you should be sure all author names and affiliations are correct (usually, there is at least one error). Make sure all the authors who worked on the manuscript are included! Additionally, the production team may have questions about the manuscript that you will have the opportunity to respond to on this PDF document. Be sure to double-triple-check this document! Failure to catch errors here will force you to publish a corrigendum along with the manuscript on PubMed, which will be viewed indefinitely! This is not the worst thing in the world to happen, but it would be nice to avoid it. After proofing your article, it should appear online and be indexed in PubMed within weeks.

Post-Publication Issues

Once the manuscript is officially published, post-publication correspondence can be used for a multitude of different reasons. We will discuss some of these reasons here. Many times, other investigators from other studies may be performing their own studies and request data from your study through the corresponding author's address. Additional issues can be brought up, such as having errors in small parts of your paper. If small enough, it is best to just submit a correction to the journal, and this will be published as a corrigendum similar to the author issue mentioned above. A corrigendum will be viewed indefinitely; therefore, future researchers will be able to view the incorrect version of your paper along with the submitted correction afterward. Therefore, it is better to correct it the first time, although this may not always be the case — accidents do happen. However, when someone, after publication, notices many errors, this is where it gets tricky. In cases where the overall paper is unsalvageable, such as a survival analysis for a type of cancer where the entire model is now flawed and incorrect, or, alternatively, if the paper was found to be almost completely taken from another investigator due to ethical concerns, this could warrant a retraction. A retracted publication is not good for any investigator — this means that there was a flaw found in the publication that was not reparable. In these cases, the paper is marked as retracted in the journal and on PubMed. An additional retraction notice will also be published stating why the publication was retracted. This is rare, but it does happen. To come to this point is generally a discussion between the authors and the editors of the journal. Please do your best to make sure this does not happen to you!

Copyright

Once accepted for publication, your manuscript, comprising your writing, figures, and tables, belongs to the journal if it is a subscription journal. Therefore, if you would like to use these figures again for another work, you have to request permission to use this material again — once a journal accepts your work, it is no longer your material and is the copyright of the journal. Terms vary widely with different journals. Some journals encourage authors to share the final published manuscript publicly, while others do not. Some journals make their work free and open publicly for one year and then revert to a fee. Before widely disseminating any of your publications, it is always important to check the journal's terms and conditions before dissemination.

Part VI
Additional Topics

25 Intellectual Property

In medical school, there is very little education in intellectual property associated with research findings, even though the medical commercial industry represents approximately 17.6% of commercial business in the United States.[1] If you have an idea from your research topics, how would you carry this to market? How would you submit for a patent for your new idea or technology? In this chapter, we will discuss two main routes you can take to obtain intellectual property for your ideas. This would include using an institutional technology ventures program at your local institution in addition to submitting a patent yourself to the United States Patent and Trade Office.

What is a Patent?

A patent is a protection issued by the United States government to an inventor to protect an invention from being reproduced by another entity.[2] This patent has different lengths of effectiveness, depending on what type of patent is issued; however, a patent can generally be considered to last 20 years after the invention.[2]

First, there are two types of patents to be aware of when considering these for your ideas. The first is a **provisional patent**, which can be pursued for your idea and lasts up to one year in length. These patents are not examined by the patent office and can be thought of as a placeholder once you come up with an idea. This 1-year protection can be used to develop your idea and solidify the design before issuing a **non-provisional patent**, which would last the full 20 years.[3]

To be qualified to receive patent protection, an idea must fall into one of the four following categories: processes, machines, manufactures, and compositions of matter.[4] In an introductory healthcare book like this, we will most likely be talking about the first three types. Therefore, if you have an idea for a specific data analytic algorithm, data analytic platform, or other process, this would be patentable. If you have an idea for a physical mechanical engineering device you are studying in school, this is also patentable.[3]

Inventors

In general and legally, the position of inventors does not matter, unlike article publications. The primary inventor is listed first, as this patent would be referenced with this person's last name. For example, a patent would be referenced as "Last name *et al.*" when referencing a patent. After the primary inventor, additional inventors are typically listed in alphabetical order.[5]

Parts of a Patent

There are four main parts to complete a patent. See Appendix 4 for an example of an entire submitted patent for a "stick" that is used as a dog toy.

First, there is an abstract, which is a brief summary of an invention. This describes the novelty of the intellectual property being protected. Second, there is a brief drawing of the invention. This can be handwritten or professionally performed and will typically consist of many different views of the patented object, along with a numbering scheme to correlate this picture with the claims of the patent. Third, there is the background of the invention, which is a more in-depth description of the problem the invention is trying to solve. Finally, a summary portion is completed that has the annotation of a listing of claims on the drawing describing the invention. This is arguably one of the most important parts of the patent because it lists all of the covered areas and features of the new invention. These claims are typically numerically schemed and can be correlated with the patent illustration.

How to Pursue a Patent

There are two main pathways to pursuing a patent. The first step is pursuing patent protection through your institutional tech ventures program. This is suggested as the appropriate method for pursuing patent protection if you have never completed this process before in the past. In this process, the institution will have a staff of intellectual property attorneys and writing staff who can complete a draft of the patent on your behalf. This would be free to you as the inventor. However, the institution will typically take a portion of your profit. This percentage withheld by the institution can range from 20% to 100%. Ultimately, however, if you are new to the process, it is better to pursue this through the Tech Transfer department so that you can learn the complete process before doing it on your own. The Tech Transfer department typically also helps with licensing (having third-party companies pay to use your intellectual property) and overall developing your product as well.

If you do attempt to complete this on your own, applications can be typed or written and submitted to the United States Patent and Trademark Office online through the online application system.[6] To complete a non-provisional patent application, you would need to be a registered pro-se inventor. This often has the requirements of mailing in your documents and can take a few months to complete. The benefit of this route is that you get to retain your percentage of revenue from your intellectual property for yourself.

When Deciding to Pursue Patent Protection

Multiple different variables should be used when deciding to pursue patent protection. For example, in a rapidly changing field with innovative technology changing monthly, weekly, or daily, the amount of time and money to pursue patent protection may not be worth the squeeze. This can be true for rapidly developing areas, such as computer programs, artificial intelligence, and devices outside the medical space that do not require FDA approval. However, if you have a medical device that takes years to get approved by the FDA, this would be a worthwhile device to pursue patent protection, as it takes a long time to get this approved and would be less likely to become outdated during the years of patent protection.

References

1. Center for Medicare & Medicaid Services. Historical. 2024. Accessed at: https://www.cms.gov/data-research/statistics-trends-and-reports/national-health-expenditure-data/historical#:~:text=Pages%20in%20this%20section&text=The%20National%20Health%20Expenditure%20Accounts,-For%20additional%20information%2C%20see%20below.
2. United States Patent and Trademark Office. Patent essentials. Accessed at: https://www.uspto.gov/patents/basics/essentials#:~:text=How%20long%20is%20a%20patent,may%20be%20extended%20or%20adjusted.

3. Harvard Business School. Fast answers. May 8, 2024. Accessed at: https://asklib.library.hbs.edu/faq/267581#:~:text=A%20nonprovisional%20patent%20application%20is,competitive%20advantage%20in%20early%20stage.

4. United States Patent and Trademark Office. 2106 patent subject matter eligibility. 2019. Accessed at: https://www.uspto.gov/web/offices/pac/mpep/s2106.html#:~:text=THE%20FOUR%20CATEGORIES-,35%20U.S.C.,reach%20of%20patentable%20subject%20matter.

5. University of Washington. Inventorship. 2024. Accessed at: https://comotion.uw.edu/intellectual-property/patents/inventorship/#:~:text=The%20order%20of%20the%20inventors,to%20when%20referencing%20the%20patent.

6. United States Patent and Trademark Office. Applying for patents. Accessed at: https://www.uspto.gov/patents/basics/apply.

26 Mastering Grant Writing for Research Success

Securing funding is often a critical milestone in a researcher's career, enabling one to launch pilot projects, conduct advanced experiments, collaborate across institutions, and ultimately bring new discoveries to light. Yet, the process of writing a grant can be both exhilarating and daunting. A strong proposal must not only present your research idea convincingly but also demonstrate feasibility, budget alignment, and alignment with the mission of the funding agency.

This chapter provides a detailed guide to developing compelling grant proposals. We will explore:

- How to identify suitable funding sources and mechanisms
- Crafting essential sections of a grant application (e.g., Specific Aims, Budget, Significance)
- Techniques for building a persuasive narrative
- Navigating the review process and common pitfalls
- Best practices for resubmission and long-term grant-seeking success.

Whether you are an early-career investigator or a seasoned professional seeking to expand your funding portfolio, this chapter offers insights and tools to help you write winning proposals.

Understanding the Funding Landscape

Types of Funding Sources

There are several government agencies that provide opportunities for research funding. These include the National Institutes of Health (NIH) in the United States, the Medical Research Council (MRC) in the United Kingdom, the Canadian Institutes of Health Research (CIHR) in Canada, and the European Research Council (ERC) in the European Union and the United States, among others.[1,2] These sources typically fund projects aligned with national research priorities, offering substantial budgets but with highly competitive review processes (Fig. 26.1).

The next category of funding entities would be foundations and non-profits. Examples of these entities include the Bill & Melinda Gates Foundation, the Robert Wood Johnson Foundation, or disease-specific organizations such as the American Heart Association. These organizations often focus on particular diseases, population health concerns, or novel interventions. They may have less administrative red tape than government agencies but can be just as competitive.

Professional societies like the American College of Cardiology or the Society for Neuroscience may offer grants, fellowships, or travel awards. These entities typically provide smaller grants aimed at seed funding or early-career investigators.

Industry and corporate partnerships will allow funding for research that aligns with their product pipeline and strategic goals. These can include pharmaceutical companies, biotech firms, or technology corporations. Intellectual property and conflict-of-interest considerations can be more complex, requiring careful negotiation and transparency.

Internal/institutional grants may be an option, as many universities or hospitals offer intramural grants or pilot awards to

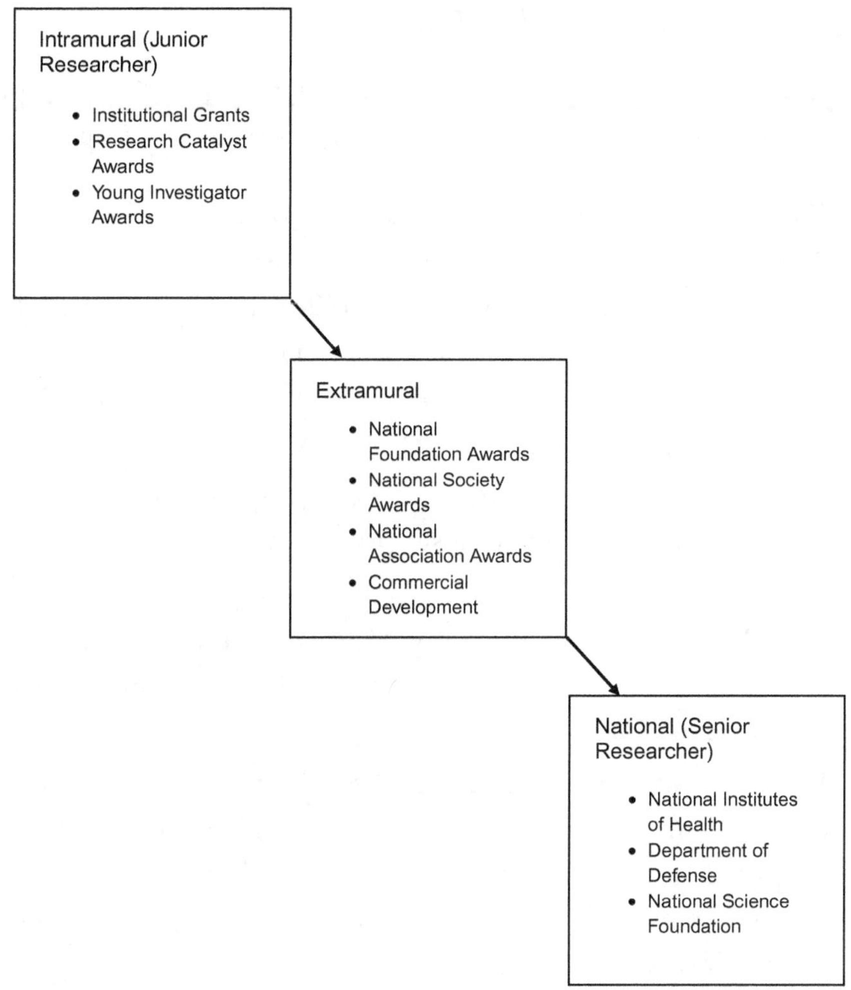

Fig. 26.1. Timeline for grant writing throughout a career.

foster early-stage research. These may have lower maximum budgets than major external grants but are typically less competitive and a good stepping stone.

International collaborations and consortia support global or multinational funding (e.g., World Health Organization, global research consortia) may back transnational projects with a broad impact. These often require multidisciplinary, multi-country collaborations, and a strong justification for cross-border research.

Grant Funding Mechanisms

Within each funding source, different mechanisms exist to support various research stages and investigator profiles. Key examples:

- **Career development grants** (K awards, Fellowships)
  - Often aimed at early-stage scientists transitioning to independence (e.g., NIH K99/R00 in the United States). Emphasizes mentorship plans, training objectives, and a trajectory toward becoming a fully independent researcher.

- **Project-based grants** (R01, R21, R03)
  - R01-like grants: Larger-scale, multi-year projects that demand a robust hypothesis, preliminary data, and detailed methodology.
  - R21 or R03: Smaller, exploratory, or pilot grants that support high-risk, high-reward ideas, and preliminary data collection.

- **Program project or center grants** (P series)
  - Multi-component projects, often involving multiple principal investigators and subprojects, designed to address a complex problem or theme. Requires strong institutional infrastructure and leadership.

- **Pilot grants or seed funds**
  - Provide smaller amounts of funding intended to generate preliminary data or test new ideas. Crucial stepping-stones for securing larger external grants.

- **Infrastructure or equipment grants**
  - Focused on acquiring or upgrading core research facilities (e.g., lab equipment, biobanks). Usually require demonstrating broad institutional impact and a sustainability plan.

Laying the Foundation: From Idea to Proposal

Matching Your Idea to the Right Mechanism

When attempting to find the right mechanism, you have to consider several aspects. First, you need to consider the scope and stage of your research. Do you need a smaller grant for early proof-of-concept, or are you ready for a large-scale R01-type project? Some grants cover just 1–2 years, while others can extend to 5 years or more. Early-career researchers may target fellowships or K-type awards; established investigators might pursue R01 or P-series grants. Finally, you need to consider the research priorities of the potential funders. Align your proposal with the agency's stated mission, strategic goals, and current funding priorities.

Preliminary Data and Team Readiness

It is important to consider the preliminary data you have obtained for your project.

This strengthens your credibility and demonstrates feasibility. Even a small pilot study or proof-of-concept experiments can significantly bolster your proposal. It is important to balance preliminary data with the potential for novelty. While robust data can be persuasive, showing moderate but promising pilot results can also highlight the novelty and risk-reward balance of your project.

It is important to build a team with diverse expertise. Reviewers look for synergy — biostatisticians, clinicians, basic scientists, or engineers may all be needed, depending on your question. It is also important to have a strong system of mentors and collaborators. Letters of support from recognized leaders in the field bolster your application's impact and feasibility.

Key Components of a Strong Grant Application

Although formatting requirements differ across agencies, several elements commonly appear in grant proposals:

Specific Aims (or Objectives)

Provide a concise, high-level overview of the project's main research goals or hypotheses.

Typically limited to 1 page (e.g., NIH format). This section is often the first section that reviewers read — so clarity and impact are critical.

To create the structure, you need to provide an introduction/context paragraph. Briefly state the problem and why it matters (clinical significance, knowledge gap). After this, you should provide an overall hypothesis: Offer a bold, central statement. Next, describe specific aims. Number them (usually 2–3), each with a specific question and expected outcomes. Lastly, you should state a lasting impact. Close with a statement on how successful your completion of aims will advance the field.

Background and Significance

Demonstrate a deep understanding of relevant literature and highlight why your question remains unanswered. Justify the need for your proposed study and summarize key studies or data. Avoid burying reviewers in excessive detail — focus on what is most relevant to your aims. Identify gaps by explicitly showing how your work addresses overlooked aspects, resolves conflicting findings or applies a novel method. Emphasize public health or societal relevance.

Preliminary Data (If Required or Applicable)

Provides evidence that your approach is valid and feasible and that you or your team have the expertise to carry out the proposed research. For content, provide the essential figures/tables: Graphs or images demonstrating pilot results, feasibility, or proof-of-concept. Describe your methods by having summaries of how preliminary data were obtained, focusing on reliability and significance. Have a narrative of evolution by showing how early findings shaped your current hypothesis or methodology.

Research Plan or Methods

Outline in detail how you will achieve each aim, from experimental design to data analysis.

Be sure that this section contains the following core elements:

- **Design and approach**
  - Specify the overall study design (e.g., randomized controlled trial, cohort study, *in vitro* experiments).
  - Justify the sample size with power calculations, if relevant.
- **Methods**
  - Identify primary outcomes, measurement tools, software, or assays.
  - Describe procedures in sufficient detail so that reviewers can assess feasibility and rigor.
- **Data analysis**
  - Outline your plan for statistical or computational analysis.
  - Mention how you will handle confounding variables, missing data, or potential biases.

- **Potential pitfalls and alternatives**
  - Demonstrate foresight by identifying possible challenges (e.g., low recruitment, data variability) and strategies to mitigate them.

Timeline and Milestones

This section will illustrate project organization, ensuring feasibility within the grant's duration. Create a simple Gantt chart or table showing each aim's activities and approximate time windows.

Highlight major milestones (e.g., completing recruitment, finishing lab assays, writing manuscripts).

Budget and Justification

Show how requested funds directly support the research activities. Convince reviewers the budget is reasonable and is neither inflated nor unrealistically minimal.

Common budget categories include:

- Personnel: Salaries for investigators, research assistants, technicians, and statisticians.
- Equipment: Specialized instruments or software (if essential).
- Supplies: Consumables, reagents, etc.
- Travel: Conferences and site visits, if relevant.
- Facilities and administrative costs (Indirects): Handled by institution-specific rates, if allowed by the funder.

Budget justification

- Detail how each line item supports a specific aspect of the study.
- Avoid vague justifications like "miscellaneous" or "contingencies."

Letters of Support

Demonstrate institutional backing, partnerships, and external endorsements. Validate your access to populations, specialized equipment, or mentorship. Ensure letters come from genuinely engaged collaborators or mentors. Highlight what each supporting party uniquely contributes (e.g., patient recruitment site, data analysis expertise).

Biosketch and Other Support Forms

- **Biosketch:** Most grants will request an official NIH Biosketch (see Appendix 4) (OMB No. 0925-0001 and 0925-0002). This is a document with strict criteria that can range from 1 to 5 pages.[3] This is a brief overview of a researcher's previous experiences and current work. It is important to use the most updated document, as this worksheet is reformatted every few years by the National Institutes of Health.
- **Other support:** Additionally, grants will oftentimes require an NIH "Other Support" form (see Appendix 5)(PHS 398). This describes the researcher's support for other work.[4] The primary goal of this document is to make sure that the researcher is overfunded with many projects occurring at one time.

Crafting a Compelling Narrative

Establishing Significance and Innovation

Tie your research to real-world needs (patient care, policy gaps, technological advances). Clarify the ramifications of success — how might your work change guidelines, technologies, or future studies? Emphasize unique approaches: novel application of a known method, cross-disciplinary teamwork, or technology adaptation to an underexplored domain. Position your project as both grounded (feasible) and forward thinking.

Use Clear, Concise Language

Grant reviewers often read dozens of proposals under time pressure. Make their job easier by writing in a direct, logical style. Add headings and subheadings, which will help reviewers navigate. Use short paragraphs to keep text accessible. Minimize jargon and define specialized terms or acronyms, especially for cross-disciplinary review panels. Use a logical flow to build from broad context to specific methods — each section should seamlessly connect to the next.

Achieving Cohesion

Your aims, background, methods, and budget must align. A mismatch (e.g., an ambitious aim with insufficient budget) can raise red flags. Cross-reference among multiple documents. For example, mention "Aim 2" in both the methods and timeline for clarity. Review for consistency by ensuring there are no contradictory statements about the sample size or methodology across sections. Be sure that each item discussed on each document is consistent throughout all documents. Use a thematic through-line by reinforcing the central hypothesis or main goal in every major section.

Navigating the Review Process

Understanding Grant Review Criteria

Common criteria:

- **Significance:** Does it address an important problem or critical barrier in the field?

- **Investigator(s):** Are the PI and team well-qualified?
- **Innovation:** How novel are the concepts, methods, or interventions?
- **Approach:** Is the design sound, with robust statistics and feasible methods?
- **Environment:** Does the institution or setting facilitate success?

Peer Review Panels

You can expect multiple reviewers with relevant but diverse expertise, each scoring or rating your proposal based on the agency's criteria. An overall discussion leading to a priority score or funding recommendation.

Communicating with Program Officers (If Applicable)

Program officers can guide you on alignment with the funding agency's priorities, the competitiveness of your idea, or ways to improve your proposal. Be sure to have early engagement by reaching out before submission if the agency allows or encourages it. Have a constructive dialog by asking clarifying questions and being open to feedback, but keep communications professional and succinct.

Packaging and Submitting the Application

Agencies often have strict page limits, font requirements, and electronic submission protocols. Missing a detail (e.g., references exceeding a page limit) can lead to administrative rejection.

Internal Reviews and Feedback

Ask colleagues or mentors to read the proposal critically. Many universities have grant review offices or "mock study sections" to give feedback. Typos or poorly structured sentences can overshadow strong ideas.

Final Checks

Ensure your resources listed in the budget are in line with your stated aims. Be sure that figures and tables are clear, e.g., high-quality graphics reinforce your arguments effectively. Submit early, if possible, to troubleshoot technical issues with online portals (e.g., Grants.gov, Research.gov, or agency-specific platforms).

After Submission: What Next?

Scenario 1: Your Grant is Funded

- **Negotiations:** Sometimes, budget or scope modifications are requested before final approval.
- **Implementation:** Begin work promptly, track milestones, and maintain strong communication with the sponsor.

Scenario 2: Your Grant is Not Funded

- **Review feedback:** Analyze critiques closely. Identify patterns — did the reviewers question feasibility, significance, or clarity?
- **Resubmission:** Address concerns methodically. Revise aims if needed, strengthen methodology, and highlight any new preliminary data.

- **Alternative funding:** Keep an eye out for other agencies or calls for proposals that might be a better fit.

Building a Track Record

Securing a grant (even a small one) strengthens your CV and credibility for future applications. Funders often look for consistency and a track record of high-quality publications or outputs. Show productivity with pilot data, conference abstracts, or journal articles. Properly cite your grant in any publications or presentations. Successful collaborators often open doors to bigger or multi-institutional grants.

Common Pitfalls and How to Avoid Them

- **Overly ambitious scope**
  - Reviewers may doubt feasibility. Focus on a few well-defined aims with a clear path.

- **Weak preliminary data**
  - Even small pilot data or a strong rationale can help establish feasibility.

- **Poorly justified budget**
  - Misaligned or unclear budget requests erode reviewer confidence.

- **Ignoring reviewer feedback**
  - For resubmissions, failing to address prior critiques typically leads to repeated rejection.

- **Lack of clarity**
  - Vague methods, tangential aims, or inconsistent writing hamper the overall impact.

Conclusion

Grant writing is both an art and a science — a well-crafted proposal weaves together rigorous methodology, compelling significance, careful budgeting, and a clear demonstration of your team's expertise. Success depends not only on the merits of your research idea but also on how effectively you communicate its promise.

Know your funder: Tailor each proposal to the priorities and requirements of the funding agency or organization.

Plan thoroughly: Start early, gather strong preliminary data if possible, and refine each section for maximum clarity.

Collaborate wisely: Engage mentors, statisticians, technical experts, and community partners to fill expertise gaps and strengthen feasibility.

Persist and evolve: Rejections are common. Use reviewer feedback to revise proposals, gather more data, or pivot to new funding opportunities.

By mastering the grant writing process, you will not only secure essential resources but also sharpen your research focus and build lasting partnerships. Over time, these skills can significantly accelerate your career, fuel scientific discoveries, and contribute to meaningful advancements in healthcare, technology, education, or any other field.

References

1. National Institutes of Health. Grants & funding. 2024. Accessed at: https://grants.nih.gov/.

2. Grants.gov. U.S. Department of Defense (DOD). 2024. Accessed at: https://www.grants.gov/learn-grants/grant-making-agencies/u-s-department-of-defense-dod.

3. National Institutes of Health. Biosketch format pages, instructions, and samples. Accessed at: https://grants.nih.gov/grants-process/write-application/forms-directory/biosketch.

4. National Institutes of Health. Other support. Accessed at: https://grants.nih.gov/grants-process/write-application/forms-directory/other-support.

Additional Recommended Readings and Resources

- European Research Council (ERC) Funding & Grants: erc.europa.eu
- Foundation Center: foundationcenter.org
- Grant Writing Basics: *The Grant Application Writer's Workbook* by Russell & Morrison
- National Science Foundation (NSF) Funding: nsf.gov/funding/
- NIH Grants & Funding Site: grants.nih.gov

27 Ending Thoughts

The information contained in this book should be of significant assistance for you to go forward with completing your medical studies. If you read this book, you should have a basic understanding on how to formulate ideas, acquire data, analyze data, and publish your results.

Given all of this information, however, this book is not designed to replace mentorship by faculty members. This is only intended to be an adjunct in the learning process. Everyone needs mentorship, and in no way, shape, or form are we advocating you not to find a mentor, no matter what situation you are in. If you are in a small medical school without many mentors, attempt to collaborate with potential mentors at other institutions. Some mentors are very passionate about teaching others and are willing to help people from different institutions. This is especially true if you have no home program for your intended specialty. Learning from others who are more experienced is paramount in the medical education process. One avenue for finding mentors is attending local and national conferences for your medical specialty. Many of these conferences have young professionals sections specifically designed for networking. Additionally, many national specialty associations have direct programs where you can register online and be placed with a mentor near your geographic location.

If you found this book helpful, please feel free to review this book online at Amazon.com, Barnes & Noble, or another bookselling entity. Additionally, if you have any comments or suggestions for improvement, please list these in the online reviews.

Did we miss something?
See any errors?

Please feel free to leave a review on Amazon.com or Worldscientific.com for thoughts and corrections on future content.

Have you read?
More publications by the same authors

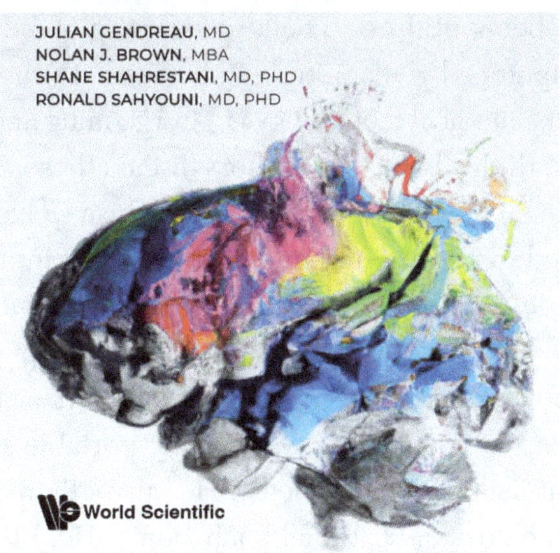

What is machine learning? What is the current state of prosthetics in healthcare? Can scientists cure paralysis? Are supercomputers composed of human DNA real? These are all questions contemplated by both highly educated biomedical engineers and individuals without formal scientific training who have simple interests in medicine. Technology, undoubtedly, has given rise to advancements in many diverse areas of our lives today. It has led to improvements in the ways we complete business transactions, the ways we use social media to connect with others, and the methods we use to treat patients in medicine. This is especially true when examining neuroscience approaches in technology, otherwise known as neuroengineering. Concepts such as machine learning and artificial intelligence will one day assist practitioners in making more accurate and superior medical diagnoses. Novel prosthetics are currently being devised, utilizing intracranial brain computer interfaces to recreate patient thoughts for controlling these prosthetics. Supercomputers, composed of human genetic material, are being utilized to make processing speeds faster than current computers by magnitudes of speed. With all of these advancements, medical technology is a burgeoning and interesting area of study. In this book, the authors discuss these technological advancements in healthcare in 14 comprehensive chapters specifically designed to be read and understood by any individual interested in learning more about technology in medicine. Co-author Nolan Brown has over 100 peer-reviewed publications in the neurosurgical and neuroengineering literature. Dr Shane Shahrestani, MD, PhD, participated in the world's first portable stroke detection device utilizing magnetic fields. He currently has NIH grant funding for the device. Dr Ronald Sahyouni, MD, PhD, has novel work in myoelectric prosthetic devices. From discussing topics such as creating the first human cyborgs to discussing topics on humankind's first attempt at curing paralysis, this book takes an informative approach to educate interested individuals regardless of their educational background.

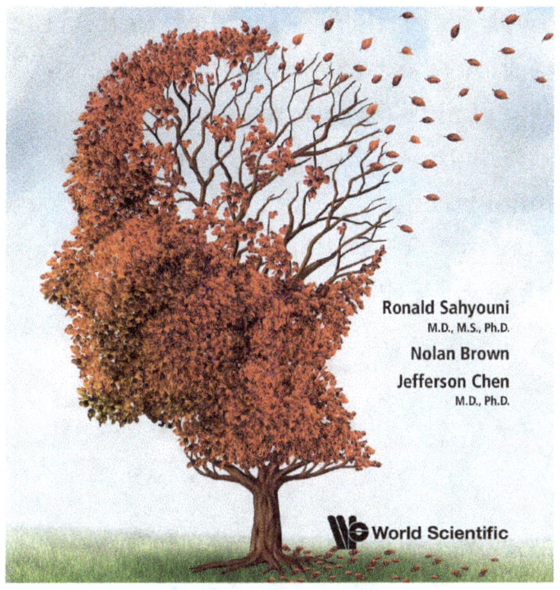

This book aims to present, educate, and inform individuals about Alzheimer's disease in a comprehensive manner. Its scope ranges from the discovery of the disease, epidemiology, and basic biological principles underlying it to advanced stem cell therapies used in the treatment of Alzheimer's. It adopts a "global" perspective on Alzheimer's disease and includes epidemiological data and science from countries around the world.

Alzheimer's disease is a rapidly growing problem seen in every country. This is the first and only comprehensive book to cover Alzheimer's disease and includes the most updated literature and scientific progress in the field of dementia and Alzheimer's disease research. Most books on the market that focus on Alzheimer's disease are targeted at caregivers with practical advice on how to deal with loved ones with the disease. This book is instead a comprehensive and popular science book that can be read by anyone with an interest in learning more about the disease. Dr Jefferson Chen, MD, PhD, co-author, participated in the world's first surgical clinical trial using shunts to treat Alzheimer's disease. His first-hand involvement in a clinical trial for patients with Alzheimer's disease and experience treating Normal Pressure Hydrocephalus (NPH), which is commonly misdiagnosed as Alzheimer's disease, lends a unique perspective. This book will appeal to a wide audience, regardless of their scientific or educational background.

Appendix 1: Preferred Reporting Items for Systematic Review and Meta-Analyses

TITLE		
Title	1	Identify the report as a systematic review.
ABSTRACT		
Abstract	2	See the PRISMA 2020 for Abstracts checklist.
INTRODUCTION		
Rationale	3	Describe the rationale for the review in the context of existing knowledge.
Objectives	4	Provide an explicit statement of the objective(s) or question(s) the review addresses.
METHODS		
Eligibility criteria	5	Specify the inclusion and exclusion criteria for the review and how studies were grouped for the syntheses.
Information sources	6	Specify all databases, registers, websites, organizations, reference lists, and other sources searched or consulted to identify studies. Specify the date when each source was last searched or consulted.
Search strategy	7	Present the full search strategies for all databases, registers, and websites, including any filters and limits used.

(Continued)

(Continued)

Selection process	8	Specify the methods used to decide whether a study met the inclusion criteria of the review, including how many reviewers screened each record and each report retrieved, whether they worked independently, and, if applicable, details of automation tools used in the process.
Data collection process	9	Specify the methods used to collect data from reports, including how many reviewers collected data from each report, whether they worked independently, any processes for obtaining or confirming data from study investigators, and, if applicable, details of automation tools used in the process.
Data items	10a	List and define all outcomes for which data were sought. Specify whether all results that were compatible with each outcome domain in each study were sought (e.g., for all measures, time points, analyses), and, if not, the methods used to decide which results to collect.
	10b	List and define all other variables for which data were sought (e.g., participant and intervention characteristics, funding sources). Describe any assumptions made about any missing or unclear information.
Study risk of bias assessment	11	Specify the methods used to assess the risk of bias in the included studies, including details of the tool(s) used, how many reviewers assessed each study and whether they worked independently, and, if applicable, details of automation tools used in the process.
Effect measures	12	Specify the effect measure(s) for each outcome (e.g., risk ratio, mean difference) used in the synthesis or presentation of results.
Synthesis methods	13a	Describe the processes used to decide which studies were eligible for each synthesis (e.g., tabulating the study intervention characteristics and comparing against the planned groups for each synthesis (item #5)).

(Continued)

	13b	Describe any methods required to prepare the data for presentation or synthesis, such as the handling of missing summary statistics or data conversions.
	13c	Describe any methods used to tabulate or visually display the results of individual studies and syntheses.
	13d	Describe any methods used to synthesize results and provide a rationale for the choice(s). If meta-analysis was performed, describe the model(s)/method(s) to identify the presence and extent of statistical heterogeneity, and the software package(s) used.
	13e	Describe any methods used to explore possible causes of heterogeneity among study results (e.g., subgroup analysis, meta-regression).
	13f	Describe any sensitivity analyses conducted to assess the robustness of the synthesized results.
Reporting bias assessment	14	Describe any methods used to assess the risk of bias due to missing results in a synthesis (arising from reporting biases).
Certainty assessment	15	Describe any methods used to assess certainty (or confidence) in the body of evidence for an outcome.
RESULTS		
Study selection	16a	Describe the results of the search and selection process, from the number of records identified in the search to the number of studies included in the review, ideally using a flow diagram.
	16b	Cite studies that might appear to meet the inclusion criteria but which were excluded, and explain why they were excluded.
Study characteristics	17	Cite each included study and present its characteristics.
Risk of bias in studies	18	Present assessments of risk of bias for each included study.

(Continued)

(Continued)

Results of individual studies	19	For all outcomes, present for each study: (a) summary statistics for each group (where appropriate) and (b) an effect estimate and its precision (e.g., confidence/credible interval), ideally using structured tables or plots.
Results of syntheses	20a	For each synthesis, briefly summarize the characteristics and risk of bias among contributing studies.
	20b	Present results of all statistical syntheses conducted. If meta-analysis was done, present for each the summary estimate and its precision (e.g., confidence/credible interval) and measures of statistical heterogeneity. If comparing groups, describe the direction of the effect.
	20c	Present results of all investigations of possible causes of heterogeneity among study results.
	20d	Present results of all sensitivity analyses conducted to assess the robustness of the synthesized results.
Reporting biases	21	Present assessments of risk of bias due to missing results (arising from reporting biases) for each synthesis assessed.
Certainty of evidence	22	Present assessments of certainty (or confidence) in the body of evidence for each outcome assessed.
DISCUSSION		
Discussion	23a	Provide a general interpretation of the results in the context of other evidence.
	23b	Discuss any limitations of the evidence included in the review.
	23c	Discuss any limitations of the review processes used.
	23d	Discuss the implications of the results for practice, policy, and future research.
OTHER INFORMATION		
Registration and protocol	24a	Provide registration information for the review, including the register name and registration number, or state that the review was not registered.

(Continued)

	24b	Indicate where the review protocol can be accessed or state that a protocol was not prepared.
	24c	Describe and explain any amendments to information provided at registration or in the protocol.
Support	25	Describe sources of financial or non-financial support for the review and the role of the funders or sponsors in the review.
Competing interests	26	Declare any competing interests of review authors.
Availability of data, code and other materials	27	Report which of the following are publicly available and where they can be found: template data collection forms; data extracted from included studies; data used for all analyses; analytic code; any other materials used in the review.

Reference: Page MJ, McKenzie JE, Bossuyt PM, Boutron I, Hoffmann TC, Mulrow CD, *et al*. The PRISMA 2020 statement: An updated guideline for reporting systematic reviews. *British Medical Journal*. 2021; **372**: n71. doi: 10.1136/bmj.n71

Appendix 2: Example of Manuscript Formatting

1   Title: **Endovascular versus Open Microsurgical Intervention** for **Dural Arteriovenous**
2   **Fistulas of the Craniovertebral** Junction**: A Systematic Review of the Current Evidence**

3
4   Nolan J. Brown BS[1]; Cathleen C. Kuo BS[2]; Michael T. Lawton MD[3]

5   [1]Department of Neurological Surgery, University of California, San Diego, CA
6   [2]Department of Neurosurgery, University at Buffalo, Buffalo, NY
7   [3]Departement of Neurosurgery, Barrow Neurological Institute, St. Joseph's Hospital and Medical
8   Center, Phoenix, AZ

9
10   **Running Title**: ENDOVASCULAR EMBOLIZATAION VERSUS MICROSURGERY: CCJ
11   dAVFs
12
13
14   **Correspondence:**
15   Michael T. Lawton, M.D.
16   Department of Neurosurgery
17   Barrow Neurological Institute
18   Email: Michael.lawton@barrowbrainandspine.com | Phone: 855-977-9496
19

20   *Abstract Word Count*: 293
21   *Manuscript Word Count*: 4169
22   *Figure and Table Count*: 4
23   *Reference Count*: 114
24

25

26

27

28

29

30

31

32

33

34

35

36

37

Nolan Brown-M24
Deleted:

Brown, Nolan (Medical Student)
Deleted: Conflicts of Interest: None
Funding: None
Disclosures: None
Previous Submission: None

Nolan Brown-M24
Deleted:

Brown, Nolan (Medical Student)
Deleted: *Disclosures: None*
Financial Support: None

Brown, Nolan (Medical Student)
Formatted: Font: Not Bold, Italic

Brown, Nolan (Medical Student)
Deleted: 375

Brown, Nolan (Medical Student)
Formatted: Font: Not Bold, Italic

Brown, Nolan (Medical Student)
Formatted: Font: Italic

Brown, Nolan (Medical Student)
Formatted: Font: Italic

Brown, Nolan (Medical Student)
Formatted: Font: Not Bold, Italic

Brown, Nolan (Medical Student)
Formatted: Font: Italic

Brown, Nolan (Medical Student)
Formatted: Font: Italic

Brown, Nolan (Medical Student)
Formatted: Font: Not Bold, Italic

Brown, Nolan (Medical Student)
Deleted:

Brown, Nolan (Medical Student)
Deleted:

50   Abstract

51   **Introduction**

52   Dural arteriovenous fistulas of the craniocervical junction (CCJ dAVFs) are challenging to treat

53   due to their heterogeneous angioarchitecture and proximity to critical brainstem

54   neurovasculature. As no consensus exists regarding their treatment, the objective of the present

55   study is to explore the safety and efficacy of endovascular versus microsurgical treatment of CCJ

56   dAVFs.

57

58   **Methods**

59   We conducted a three-database scoping review according to PRISMA-ScR guidelines. Inclusion

60   criteria were defined as follows: patients with CCJ dAVFs who were treated with microsurgery

61   or endovascular therapy and seen for follow-up at a minimum of 6 months.

62

63   **Results**

64   Of the 357 studies screened, a total of 77 reports met criteria for inclusion. Among the 195

65   patients diagnosed with CCJ dAVF, 105 (60.6 +/- 11.1 years, 77 males) were treated

66   microsurgically while 68 (56.2 +/- 13.1 years, 50 males) received endovascular therapy. When

67   compared to patients who underwent surgery, patients who received endovascular therapy were

68   younger (p=0.015) and more likely to present with tinnitus (p=0.001). For both treatment groups,

69   the most common finding on presentation was subarachnoid hemorrhage (SAH). In similar

70   fashion, myelopathy and quadriparesis were both equally pervasive and fairly common on

71   presentation in both groups (p=0.116 and 0.254). Surgical and radiographic outcomes indicate

72   that both open microsurgery and endovascular therapy are adequate treatment modalities for CCJ

73   dAVF. However, endovascular therapy is associated with a significantly higher rate of

74   permanent neurological deficits post-intervention (p=0.036).

75

76   **Conclusion**

77   Treatment of CCJ dAVFs with endovascular embolization has proven challenging in previous

78   studies. As such, microsurgical intervention remains a viable option for many patients receiving

79   treatment for CCJ dAVF, as rates of permanent neurologic deficits are higher

125 following endovascular therapy. Nonetheless, due to the rarity of CCJ dAVFs, there remains a

126 paucity of data in the literature and firm conclusions cannot yet be made.

127

128 **Abbreviations**: AVM – arteriovenous malformation; CCJ – craniocervical junction; CT –

129 computed tomography; CVJ – craniovertebral junction; DAVF – dural arteriovenous fistula; ICG

130 – indocyanine green; ICH – intracranial hemorrhage; MRI – magnetic resonance imaging; PAVF

131 – perimedullary arteriovenous fistula; PICA – posterior inferior cerebellar artery; SAH –

132 subarachnoid hemorrhage.

133

134 **Keywords**: dural AVF, craniocervical junction, craniovertebral junction, endovascular,

135 cerebrovascular, skull base, open surgery, arteriovenous fistula

136

137

138

139

140

141

142

143

144

145

146

147

148

149

150

3

155   Introduction

156   Craniocervical junction dural arteriovenous fistulas (CCJ dAVFs) are rare vascular

157   malformations of the craniovertebral junction that can be challenging to diagnose and even more

158   difficult to treat.[1] Although a small subset of CCJ dAVF patients may be asymptomatic,

159   presentations can range from acute subarachnoid hemorrhage (SAH) to chronic, progressive

160   myelopathy.[3] Therefore, these vascular malformations necessitate prompt treatment. Further

161   complicating the management of CCJ dAVFs is the fact that they possess relatively more

162   complex angioarchitecture than their intracranial, subaxial-cervical, and thoracolumbar spinal

163   counterparts, and are surrounded by complex neuroanatomic structures as well, such as low

164   cranial and upper spinal nerves and caudal brainstem.[3-6]

165   Because these malformations are particularly rare, their natural history remains unclear

166   and treatment algorithms have not yet been established. At present, the two primary approaches

167   to treatment include 1) endovascular embolization and 2) microsurgical interruption of the

168   draining vein to achieve obliteration.[1,4] Because of the rarity of CCJ dAVFs and the resulting

169   dearth of literature pertaining to treatment selection and clinical outcomes, there is little

170   comparative data available regarding the proper management of patients with this subset of

171   dAVFs. For this reason, we herein perform a scoping review of the current neurosurgical

172   literature in order to compare outcomes obtained following endovascular embolization versus

173   open microsurgical obliteration for treating dAVFs of the CCJ.

174

175   Methods

176   *Literature Search*

177   This study was prepared in accordance with the Preferred Reporting Items for Systematic

178   reviews and Meta-Analyses (PRISMA) guidelines.[9] A systematic search was performed using

179   the PubMed (National Library of Medicine), EMBASE (Elsevier), and Cochrane Library from

180   date of inception through May 2023 to identify all relevant published articles. A combination of

181   the following MeSH search terms with Boolean operators was utilized: (craniocervical OR

182   craniovertebral) AND (arteriovenous OR fistula OR AVF OR dAVF). We limited the search to

183   English language publications and human subjects. The reference lists of all included articles

184   were manually checked for further relevant studies.

185

262   *Study Selection*
263   Two reviewers screened the studies independently for inclusion, and conflicts were resolved by
264   consultation with a third reviewer. The first portion of this review process involved abstract and
265   title screening, which was followed by full-text screening to establish inclusion. Observational
266   studies (case reports, retrospective case series) were included if they reported patients with CCJ
267   dAVF who were treated with either open microsurgery or endovascular embolization, provided
268   patient-level data including indications for treatment, and presented clinical outcomes at a
269   minimum 6 months follow up. We excluded articles with no available full-text or no clear
270   description of patient presentation, treatment modalities, or clinical outcomes. Abstracts,
271   commentaries, literature reviews, cadaveric studies, animal studies, editorials, and studies not
272   available in English were excluded. To avoid repeated inclusion of the same patients, we
273   considered only the most recent article from the same author or the same institution.
274
275   *Data Extraction*
276   Using a proforma, two authors independently extracted the following data: last name of first
277   author, publication year, number of patients, sex, age, CCJ dAVF location, presenting symptoms,
278   angioarchitectural traits (arterial supply, venous drainage), use of indocyanine green (ICG) or
279   fluorescein sodium, treatment modalities, follow-up duration, clinical outcomes, radiographic
280   outcome, and treatment complications, if any.
281
282   *Risk of Bias Assessment*
283   The quality assessment of included studies was scored using the Newcastle-Ottawa Scale (NOS)
284   [10] by two independent authors.[11] Any discrepancies were settled by discussion with a third author
285   who served as final arbiter. The NOS contains 3 main components: (1) selection of study groups,
286   (2) comparability of the groups, and (3) ascertainment of the outcome of interest. A maximum
287   score of 9 points can be reached, with higher NOS scores indicating less risk of bias.
288
289   For case studies or case series included, where NOS was not an appropriate evaluative tool, the
290   tool proposed by Murad et al. was used by the two independent authors. Discrepancies were
291   settled by discussion with a third author who served as final arbiter. Domains included in this
292   evaluative took are: selection, ascertainment, causality, and reporting. With this tool, case reports

293 and series were assigned an aggregate score of eight binary questions, for a maximum score of 8,
294 which is indicative of higher methodological quality.
295
296 *Outcome Grading and Follow Up Duration*
297 Clinical outcomes were divided into four categories: improved, stable, permanent deficit, or
298 death. Patients from included studies were categorized based on longest follow-up results
299 reported in their respective studies. If a clinical outcome category was specifically mentioned
300 within the study results, the patient was given that category for our analysis. When this was not
301 the case, the authors used their best judgment by comparing pre-operative baseline symptoms to
302 postoperative symptoms, neurologic deficits, and/or any permanent changes resulting from intra-
303 or post-operative complications. When applicable, patient reported outcomes were used. If there
304 was a reduction or resolution of symptoms or deficits, patients were labeled as "improved." If
305 there was no change, they were labeled as "stable." Whereas cases where patients developed new
306 or worsening symptoms or deficits were labeled as "permanent deficit." Patients reported as
307 deceased were categorized as "death."
308   In order to accurately compare post-operative outcomes, we categorized time to last
309 follow up into four categories and compared outcomes within these groups. Short-term-
310 immediate was used when the sole follow-up occurred prior to discharge, short-term was defined
311 as post-discharge and prior to three months, medium-term was the descriptor used for the 3-12
312 month range, and long term follow up was defined as greater than 12 months.
313
314 *Statistical Analysis*
315 Descriptive statistics for continuous variables were presented as mean ± standard deviation and
316 compared using Mann-Whitney U test. For categorical variables, frequency with percentage was
317 reported, and chi-squared testing was utilized to determine the difference between groups. All
318 computations were stored in the Microsoft Excel program (Microsoft Corporation, Redmond,
319 Washington, USA), and the statistical analyses were conducted using RStudio software (version
320 1.3.1056 ©2009–2020; R Studio Inc., Boston Massachusetts, USA). A P-value <0.05 was
321 considered statistically significant. Furthermore, due to the descriptive nature of the data
322 collected for this scoping review, a meta-analysis was not performed.
323

377 Results

378 A total of 357 studies were retrieved from the three databases. Following removal of duplicates,

379 abstract screening, and full-text evaluation, 77 studies featuring 195 patients were ultimately

380 included. The PRISMA search flow diagram is presented in **Figure 1.** The mean age among all

381 patients was 59.0±12.1 years, and the mean follow-up time was 29.6±39.0 months. Regarding

382 the risk of bias assessment, the mean NOS score was 3.22±0.94, with a range of 2 to 7. With a

383 mean of 3.22 and incorporation of studies with a NOS score of 2 as a minimum, we acknowledge

384 there is high risk of bias in some of the included studies. This will be kept in mind throughout the

385 interpretation of our results. **Table 1** summarizes the baseline characteristics of the included

386 studies.

387   Of the 195 patients diagnosed with CCJ dAVF, 105 (53.8%) underwent open

388 microsurgical obliteration of the draining vein and 68 (34.9%) underwent endovascular

389 embolization (using Onyx, NBCA, or Gugliemi detachable coils) (**Table 2**). When compared to

390 patients who underwent open microsurgical treatment, patients who received endovascular

391 therapy only were younger (p=0.015) and more likely to present with tinnitus (p=0.001). For

392 both treatment groups, the most common finding on presentation was subarachnoid hemorrhage

393 (SAH), followed by myelopathy and quadriparesis.

394   With respect to utilization of indocyanine green (ICG), this visualizing agent was

395 administered in 22.9% of all microsurgical cases. Fluorescein sodium, on the other hand, was not

396 commonly administered, as its use was reported for only one patient in each of the two treatment

397 groups.

398   Surgical and radiographic outcomes indicate that both open microsurgery and

399 endovascular therapy are adequate treatment modalities for CCJ dAVF. More specifically, 92.4%

400 of patients treated microsurgically and 85.3% of patients treated via endovascular means

401 demonstrated symptomatic improvement post-intervention. Of note, endovascular therapy was

402 associated with a significantly higher rate of permanent neurological deficits post-intervention

403 (p=0.036). Namely, 23.5% of patients who underwent endovascular treatment were left with at

404 least one permanent neurological deficit, a rate roughly twice as high as the rate of permanent

405 deficits observed following microsurgical interventions (most deficits resulted from ischemic

406 complications such as brainstem infarct) (10.5%) (p=0.036). Nevertheless, no significant

419 differences were observed between the two treatment modalities with respect to rates of
420 complete symptom resolution, symptom stabilization without progression, or mortality.
421

422 Discussion
423 As a result of their rarity, unclear natural history, and complex angioarchitecture, no standard
424 treatment has yet been established for cranial dAVFs involving CCJ. With the emergence of
425 endovascular techniques over the past two decades, open microneurosurgery and endovascular
426 therapies currently represent the two broad categories of treatment for CCJ dAVFs.[12] Recently,
427 there has been an increase in the number of studies published in the neurosurgical literature
428 pertaining to treatment of dAVFs.[13-16] From these studies, we can ascertain that the main
429 advantage of endovascular treatment is its minimally invasive nature, and it has emerged as the
430 treatment of choice for most cranial dAVFs. However, this is not necessarily the case for dAVFs
431 of the CCJ, as there is currently evidence (albeit limited in quantity) to suggest otherwise. To our
432 knowledge, our scoping review adds to a small body of existing evidence that compares
433 treatment options for CCJ dAVFs. Most of the current literature regarding treatment of CCJ
434 dAVFs exists as case studies, small series, or single center retrospective reviews. We present one
435 of the largest CCJ dAVF reviews, comprised of 77 studies and 173 individual patients (105
436 treated with microsurgery and 68 with endovascular embolization only.)
437   Although cranial dAVFs can be successfully managed via endovascular techniques,
438 dAVFs located at the craniocervical junction are often angioarchitecturally different and
439 therefore may necessitate alternative surgical management. For example, the largest
440 retrospective group study available to date has suggested that microsurgical interruption is
441 superior to endovascular embolization because microsurgery appears to reduce the need for
442 retreatment and may lower the risk of ischemic complications. Overall, endovascular
443 embolization of CCJ dAVFs has demonstrated a lower success rate than microsurgery along with
444 higher morbidity. Recently, two studies directly comparing endovascular embolization versus
445 open microsurgical obliteration of CCJ dAVFs pointed toward open microsurgical interruption
446 of the venous outflow (and subsequent obliteration of the lesion) as the treatment of choice.[1,8]
447 Additionally, a multicenter group study featuring ninety-seven patients reported that better
448 treatment results were obtained with open microsurgical obliteration as compared to
449 endovascular embolization, specifically with respect to rates of retreatment, ischemic

457   complications, and overall clinical outcomes.[12] In drawing upon these results, it has been
458   suggested that open microsurgical obliteration is the treatment of choice for dAVF of the CCJ,
459   even though endovascular embolization has emerged as the first line, gold standard treatment for
460   intracranial dAVFs.
461   The results of our study echo these recent trends and findings, as our analysis
462   demonstrates that both endovascular embolization and microsurgical obliteration are effective
463   treatments for CCJ dAVF that yield similar improvements in symptomatology. However,
464   endovascular embolization does not appear to be as safe as microsurgical treatment for CCJ
465   dAVF, as it was associated with a higher rate of permanent neurological deficits post-
466   intervention. More specifically, our results indicated that 23.5% of patients who underwent
467   endovascular treatment were left with at least one permanent neurological deficit, a rate roughly
468   double that observed following microsurgical intervention. Although the theoretical risks of open
469   cranial base (and/or CVJ) surgery are much higher than those of minimally invasive
470   endovascular interventions, no significant differences in mortality were detected. In fact, though
471   it may at first defy logic, fistulae located at the CVJ may be better suited for open microsurgical
472   intervention. This is because their unique location makes them readily accessible through open
473   microsurgical access – an important factor when considering that a significant portion of these
474   malformations will present emergently with acute SAH and require timely intervention. This
475   direct and timely access provides a (relatively) facile means for performing microsurgical
476   occlusion and likely explains the high obliteration rates previously obtained via microsurgery:
477   98% on postoperative digital subtraction angiography as reported by Wang and colleagues in
478   their review of 119 cases. Furthermore, an added advantage of open microsurgery (that is not
479   made possible by endovascular methods) is the ability to directly perform test occlusion of
480   arterial feeders using mini-clips.[5] During testing, ICG angiography can be used to accurately
481   visualize the microvascular circulation. These techniques help ensure that occlusion is
482   ultraselective and specific to arterial feeders of the fistula such that inadvertent occlusion of
483   critical vascular structures supplying the nearby brainstem can be avoided.[6–8] Overall, the results
484   of our study similarly point toward the safety and efficacy of microsurgical obliteration and are
485   similar to Wang's findings in other regards. For example, Wang also described younger patient
486   age and use of microsurgery to be predictive of favorable outcomes. Of note, although not
487   addressed in the present study, Wang reported hemorrhagic presentation to be predictive of

9

488   favorable patient functional and neurological outcomes.[9] One potential explanation for this latter

489   finding is that open microsurgery would often be selected by default in the setting of an urgent

490   hemorrhage requiring emergent intervention; when pursued, open microsurgical intervention

491   could have enabled rapid identification of the source of hemorrhage and occlusion of the arterial

492   feeder. If this was indeed the case – and hemorrhagic presentation was associated with the use of

493   open microsurgical treatment – then this would further support the value of open microsurgical

494   obliteration of CCJ dAVFs.

495   In the present study, endovascular therapy (on the other hand) was found to be associated

496   with higher rates of neurological deficits post-intervention, even though it is typically favored for

497   treatment of dAVFs located outside of the CCJ. Endovascular embolization of CCJ dAVFs is

498   often not feasible due to the degree of complexity of the angioarchitecture exhibited by these

499   lesions. Even when obliteration of these complex lesions is successful, they are associated with

500   an elevated risk for recanalization and recurrence. Collectively, these findings suggest that open

501   microsurgery should be employed for the majority of CCJ dAVF cases, especially considering

502   the complex, intricate angio-architectural properties specific to these dAVFs that can make

503   endovascular manipulations, and deployment of embolic agents exceedingly risky. Thus, even

504   though endovascular treatment is less invasive, it often complicated by the presence of complex

505   anastomoses forming connections between the meningeal branches of the ascending pharyngeal,

506   vertebral, and occipital arteries.[9] These dense anastomoses create fistulae supplied by multiple

507   arterial feeders that each exhibit significant tortuosity.[9] Further complicating matters, these

508   tortuous vessels are located proximal to critical brainstem neurovasculature at the CVJ, making

509   endovascular treatment even more unwieldy. When considering these factors, it logically follows

510   that endovascular treatment is riskier because fistulae at the CVJ are so readily accessible by

511   microsurgical techniques that enable prompt and efficient obliteration.

512

513   *Complex Arteriovenous Shunt*

514   Diagnosis of CCJ dAVFs can be difficult because these vascular anomalies typically feature

515   complex vascular anatomy and can involve deep-seated regions. Their arterial feeders usually

516   stem from the meningeal branches of the vertebral artery, and occasionally from the occipital or

517   ascending pharyngeal arteries, after which they become slow flowing, tortuous vessels that are

518   not amenable to endovascular embolization. Their venous outflow involves arterialized blood

10

587   draining through the medullary vein, coronal venous plexus (toward the spinal cord) or the

588   intracranial venous network (toward the brainstem and into the cavernous sinus, inferior petrosal

589   sinus, confluence of sinuses, or cortical veins). Flow imbalances can increase intravenous

590   pressure and induce SAH, the most common diagnosis at presentation.[8,26] In some cases, venous

591   outflow can occur via the epidural or paravertebral veins.[8]

592   Adding to the anatomical complexity and lesion-to-lesion variation of CCJ dAVFs is the

593   fact that fistulas of the foramen magnum, C1, and C2 levels are considered by some to comprise

594   distinct subtypes of CCJ dAVF.[10] Any pathology located at the CCJ is both a spinal and skull

595   base pathology. Because the CCJ consists of the skull base, the atlas, and the axis, there may be

596   observable variation in characteristics between fistulas located at each of these three sites.[1,3,8,34,35]

597   For example, foramen magnum dAVFs are fed by branches of the vertebral, ascending

598   pharyngeal, occipital, and/or posterior inferior cerebellar arteries, while C1 dAVFs (most

599   common location for dAVF nidus within the CCJ) arise in the dura mater of the C1 nerve root

600   sleeve and are most commonly fed by meningeal branches of the vertebral artery. Finally, C2

601   dAVFs are distinguished by the fact that they are epidural lesions, whereas C1 and foramen

602   magnum dAVFs lie within the dura.

603

604   *CCJ dAVFs of the Atlas (C1)*

605   Although SAH is very uncommon in subaxial spinal dAVFs, it is the telltale sign of symptomatic

606   dAVF at C1.[36] Interestingly, hemorrhage may not be detected on digital subtraction angiography

607   when the vertebral artery contralateral to the dAVF is not injected with contrast.[8] Typically,

608   injection of the contralateral vertebral artery would be skipped if retrograde filling of that

609   vertebral artery to the level of the posterior inferior cerebellar artery (PICA) was observed during

610   ipsilateral vertebral artery injection.[33] This means that angiographic investigation should involve

611   injecting both vertebral arteries if SAH due to dAVF of the C1 spinal nerve is suspected.[8,37] In

612   fact, it is recommended that six-vessel angiography covering the bilateral internal and external

613   carotid arteries in addition to the bilateral vertebral arteries be performed. CT and/or MR

614   angiogram also have diagnostic utility and should suffice for detection of vascular abnormalities

615   such as dilated venous outflow. According to Iampreechakul and colleagues, however, the

616   combination of digital subtraction angiography with rotational CT angiography represents the

617   gold standard for diagnosis of C1 dAVF.[15,38] This is a potent diagnostic combination because

620 rotational CT angiography can help clarify the presence of small arterial feeders and varices that
621 might otherwise go undetected. The varices are often the source of hemorrhage as the post-shunt
622 draining vein is subject to significant hemodynamic stress resulting from high-flow drainage of
623 arterialized venous blood.[39,40] The diagnostic utility of MRI, on the other hand, extends mostly to
624 myelopathic patients, as T2-weighted images can reveal presence of swelling in the cervical
625 cord.
626
627 *Foramen Magnum dAVFs*
628 As the CCJ extends from the foramen magnum to C2, it is important to consider surgical
629 approaches as they apply to CCJ dAVF of the foramen magnum, specifically. This region
630 contains very complex anatomy with arterial supply and venous drainage involving critical
631 structures at the skull base. Arterial feeder vessels for foramen magnum dAVFs include branches
632 of the vertebral artery (muscular branches), ascending pharyngeal artery (meningeal branches),
633 occipital artery, and the meningohypophyseal trunk (dorsal meningeal branch).[41] The fistula will
634 then drain through the marginal sinus, which connects to the following venous outflow tracts: 1)
635 sigmoid sinus and jugular bulb, 2) inferior petrosal sinus (which drains to the cavernous sinus),
636 and 3) spinal perimedullary veins. Each of these venous outflow pathways can cause different
637 symptoms, for example outflow via the sigmoid sinus produces tinnitus. Orbital venous
638 congestion can result from excessive flow through the inferior petrosal to the cavernous sinus
639 and typically presents with proptosis. Furthermore, drainage into the spinal perimedullary veins
640 can cause cervical myelopathy and ultimately lead to quadriparesis.
641   Open microsurgery is optimal for treating foramen magnum dAVFs as the complicated
642 angioarchitecture of these lesions renders endovascular interventions too risky. When planning
643 the craniotomy, approach selection should prioritize access to the venous end of the fistula.
644 Typically, the midline, paramedian, or far lateral suboccipital approaches provide appropriate
645 access to dAVFs of the foramen magnum and can be combined with C1-2 laminectomy and/or
646 hemilaminectomy as needed.
647
648 *Drawbacks of Endovascular Embolization*
649 In a recent retrospective series of 111 consecutive patients with CCJ dAVFs (of which 97 were
650 included for final analysis), open surgery was performed in the majority (80%) of patients.[6]

589   Interestingly, the results of the study suggest that open microsurgical interruption and

590   obliteration yielded superior results compared to endovascular treatment. Surgical intervention

591   was associated with good outcomes and lower rates of retreatment and ischemic complications

592   than endovascular embolization.[6] The higher rates of ischemic complications seen in

593   endovascular treatment were notable because these were the complications most likely to result

594   in permanent neurological deficits (most other perioperative complications resolved or were

595   reversed by treatment). The authors posit that the higher rates of ischemic complications

596   observed in the endovascular treatment group may be related to the exceedingly complex

597   angioarchitecture of CCJ dAVFs.[6] These lesions are particularly small, complex, and therefore

598   more complicated than thoracolumbar spinal dAVFs.[24] Angiographic findings have lent evidence

599   supporting the hypothesis that these lesions are complex: namely, that CCJ dAVFs are often fed

600   by exceedingly tortuous vessels and that arteriovenous shunts can develop along critical areas

601   (including the C1-C2 nerve roots, the spinal cord and nerves, and on the intradural or extradural

602   surface of the cord).[3] Furthermore, arterial feeders of CCJ dAVFs that arise directly from the

603   vertebral artery do so at a particularly straight angle and are incredibly small and tortuous. These

604   properties lead to a high risk of embolic complications and can make it difficult to advance the

605   microcatheter to the fistula site for proper endovascular embolic treatment.[5,24,35,42]

606

607   *Evidence Supports Microsurgery Via Far Lateral Approach*

608   As our review of the literature has demonstrated, open microsurgery should generally be the

609   first-line treatment for CCJ dAVFs because it is safe, efficacious, and more effective than

610   endovascular treatment while conferring less risk for complications.[6,14,34,45] Standard surgical

611   strategy will involving interruption or disconnection of the intradural draining vein; alternatively,

612   surgical ligation of the arterial feeder can also be attempted in conjunction with venous

613   disconnection.[14]

614   In a recent multi-center prospective cohort study featuring data from 38 patients treated

615   microsurgically for CCJ dAVF at 13 high-volume cerebrovascular surgery centers, the far lateral

616   approach was used to provide access for intradural clip ligation of each high-grade fistula

617   followed by disconnection of the arterialized vein.[44] Consistent with the results of our systematic

618   review, the predominant presentations at diagnosis in this study were subarachnoid/intracranial

619   hemorrhage (47.4%) and cervical myelopathy (36.8%). A majority (84.2%) of the CCJ dAVF

Brown, Nolan (Medical Student)
Deleted: to treat

Brown, Nolan (Medical Student)
Deleted: their

Brown, Nolan (Medical Student)
Deleted: of the dura mater

692   were supplied by direct meningeal branches from the V3/4 segments of the vertebral artery.[44]

693   Endovascular therapy failed in all lesions for which it was attempted (13.2%), As such, open

694   microsurgical obliteration via far lateral craniotomy (94.7%) was used for an overwhelming

695   majority of the lesions, which were all high-grade CCJ dAVFs that were deemed ineligible for or

696   had failed endovascular treatment. The result was an angiographic cure rate of 94.7% and a

697   minimal rate of retreatment of 5.3%. Neurologic outcomes were very good, as nearly 82% of

698   patients had recovered to mRS score of 0-2 by last follow-up. Ultimately, this remains the largest

699   North American primary study to describe microsurgical treatment of CCJ dAVF, and it echoes

700   the results of our summative review of all case reports and series previously described in the

701   literature. Together, Salem's study and our systematic review lend validity to the consensus that

702   first-line treatment for CCJ dAVF is microsurgical obliteration, with little room for endovascular

703   therapy to play a role.

704   In summation, outcomes obtained using the far lateral craniotomy approach are very

705   good, with multicentric data now suggesting that complete occlusion can be achieved in roughly

706   95% of cases with a minimal procedural complication rate of 2.6%.[44] As previously mentioned,

707   the convoluted anatomy of CCJ dAVFs alone makes them difficult to detect and subsequently

708   treat through endovascular interventions; at the same time, they are the lone class of dAVFs that

709   are perfectly suited for microsurgical disconnection of the venous drainage as it exits the dura.

710   Treatment can also involve surgically ligating arterial feeders and then interrupting the venous

711   outflow. Ultimately, the benefit of the far lateral approach to treatment of CCJ dAVFs is that it

712   enables obliteration of the intradural draining vein as close to the fistula point as possible.[44]

713

714   *Limitations*

715   We acknowledge several limitations to the present study, including those inherent in the design

716   of any scoping review. These limitations include potential sources of bias such as selection bias,

717   confounding, and reporting bias. Each source of bias limits the generalizability of our findings

718   and should be kept in mind. Furthermore, the systematic review process cannot fully account for

719   the wide degree of clinical heterogeneity present among the studies selected for final inclusion.

720   Variations in study sample sizes can lead to substantial differences in statistical power from

721   study to study, further complicating efforts to pool data for statistical analysis. Unfortunately, the

722   studies identified by our systematic review were not suitable for formal meta-analysis. This

659   mostly stems from limitations involving the heterogeneity of included patients, between-study

660   differences in treatment modalities and characteristics, and variability in outcome measures and

661   reporting methods from study to study.

662

663   <u>Conclusion</u>

664   Largely due to the difficulty of detecting and diagnosing all components of the fistulae and their

665   complex angioarchitectures, treatment of dAVF of the CCJ with endovascular embolization

666   appears to be associated with a higher complication rate than microsurgical interventions,

667   sometimes resulting in permanent neurological deficits. Although there can be significant

668   complications associated with both endovascular and microsurgical strategies, open

669   microsurgery yields lower rates of permanent neurologic deficits. Therefore, due to the

670   complexity of the surrounding angioarchitecture of CCJ dAVFs, we propose that microsurgery

671   can be the optimal treatment choice when performed by highly-skilled cerebrovascular

672   neurosurgeons. Nonetheless, due to the rarity of CCJ dAVFs, there remains a paucity of data in

673   the literature (with the exception of Salem's study which reports results consistent with the

674   present review). For this reason, future studies are required so that clinicians from

675   multidisciplinary care teams (neurosurgeons and neuro-interventionalists) can best understand

676   the relationship between treatment outcomes and baseline parameters such as size of the lesion,

677   patient age, and comorbidity status when treating dAVFs of the CCJ.

678

679

680

681

682

683

684   **References**

685   1.   Wang JY, Molenda J, Bydon A, et al. Natural history and treatment of craniocervical
686   junction dural arteriovenous fistulas. *J Clin Neurosci*. Nov 2015;22(11):1701-7.
687   doi:10.1016/j.jocn.2015.05.014
688   2.   Cognard C, Gobin YP, Pierot L, et al. Cerebral dural arteriovenous fistulas: clinical and
689   angiographic correlation with a revised classification of venous drainage. *Radiology*. Mar
690   1995;194(3):671-80. doi:10.1148/radiology.194.3.7862961

814   3.   Hiramatsu M, Sugiu K, Ishiguro T, et al. Angioarchitecture of arteriovenous fistulas at
815   the craniocervical junction: a multicenter cohort study of 54 patients. *J Neurosurg*. Jun
816   2018;128(6):1839-1849. doi:10.3171/2017.3.JNS163048
817   4.   Endo T, Shimizu H, Sato K, et al. Cervical perimedullary arteriovenous shunts: a study of
818   22 consecutive cases with a focus on angioarchitecture and surgical approaches. *Neurosurgery*.
819   Sep 2014;75(3):238-49; discussion 249. doi:10.1227/NEU.0000000000000401
820   5.   Fujimoto S, Takai K, Nakatomi H, Kin T, Saito N. Three-dimensional angioarchitecture
821   and microsurgical treatment of arteriovenous fistulas at the craniocervical junction. *J Clin
822   Neurosci*. Jul 2018;53:140-146. doi:10.1016/j.jocn.2018.04.065
823   6.   Takai K, Endo T, Seki T, et al. Neurosurgical versus endovascular treatment of
824   craniocervical junction arteriovenous fistulas: a multicenter cohort study of 97 patients. *Journal
825   of Neurosurgery*. 01 Aug. 2022 2022;137(2):373-380. doi:10.3171/2021.10.Jns212205
826   7.   Takai K. Update on the Diagnosis and Treatment of Arteriovenous Fistulas at the
827   Craniocervical Junction: A Systematic Review of 92 Cases. *Journal of Neuroendovascular
828   Therapy*. 2019;13(3):125-135. doi:10.5797/jnet.oa.2018-0113
829   8.   Zhao J, Xu F, Ren J, Manjila S, Bambakidis NC. Dural arteriovenous fistulas at the
830   craniocervical junction: a systematic review. *J Neurointerv Surg*. Jun 2016;8(6):648-53.
831   doi:10.1136/neurintsurg-2015-011775
832   9.   Liberati A, Altman DG, Tetzlaff J, et al. The PRISMA statement for reporting systematic
833   reviews and meta-analyses of studies that evaluate healthcare interventions: explanation and
834   elaboration. *BMJ*. 2009;339:b2700. doi:10.1136/bmj.b2700
835   10.   Matsubara S, Toi H, Takai H, et al. Variations and management for patients with
836   craniocervical junction arteriovenous fistulas: Comparison of dural, radicular, and epidural
837   arteriovenous fistulas. *Surgical Neurology International*. 2021;12
838   11.   Wells GA, Shea B, O'Connell D, et al. The Newcastle-Ottawa Scale (NOS) for assessing
839   the quality of nonrandomised studies in meta-analyses. Oxford; 2000.
840   12.   Takai K, Endo T, Seki T, Inoue T, Koyanagi I, Mitsuhara T. Neurosurgical versus
841   endovascular treatment of craniocervical junction arteriovenous fistulas: a multicenter cohort
842   study of 97 patients. *J Neurosurg*. Dec 31 2021:1-8. doi:10.3171/2021.10.Jns212205
843   13.   Onda K, Yoshida Y, Watanabe K, Arai H, Okada H, Terada T. High cervical
844   arteriovenous fistulas fed by dural and spinal arteries and draining into a single medullary vein:
845   report of 3 cases. *J Neurosurg Spine*. Mar 2014;20(3):256-64. doi:10.3171/2013.11.SPINE13402
846   14.   Goto Y, Hino A, Shigeomi Y, Oka H. Surgical Management for Craniocervical Junction
847   Arteriovenous Fistula Targeting the Intradural Feeder. *World Neurosurg*. Dec 2020;144:e685-
848   e692. doi:10.1016/j.wneu.2020.09.041
849   15.   Kinouchi H, Mizoi K, Takahashi A, Nagamine Y, Koshu K, Yoshimoto T. Dural
850   arteriovenous shunts at the craniocervical junction. *J Neurosurg*. Nov 1998;89(5):755-61.
851   doi:10.3171/jns.1998.89.5.0755
852   16.   Kim D, Willinsky R, Geibprasert S, Krings T, Wallace C, Gentili F. Angiographic
853   characteristics and treatment of cervical spinal dural arteriovenous shunts. *American Journal of
854   Neuroradiology*. 2010;31(8):1512-1515.
855   17.   Borden JA, Wu JK, Shucart WA. A proposed classification for spinal and cranial dural
856   arteriovenous fistulous malformations and implications for treatment. *J Neurosurg*. Feb
857   1995;82(2):166-79. doi:10.3171/jns.1995.82.2.0166
858   18.   Rodesch G, Hurth M, Alvarez H, Tadie M, Lasjaunias P. Classification of spinal cord
859   arteriovenous shunts: proposal for a reappraisal--the Bicetre experience with 155 consecutive

860 patients treated between 1981 and 1999. *Neurosurgery.* Aug 2002;51(2):374-9; discussion 379-
861 80.
862 19.   Patsalides A, Knopman J, Santillan A, Tsiouris AJ, Riina H, Gobin YP. Endovascular
863 treatment of spinal arteriovenous lesions: beyond the dural fistula. *AJNR Am J Neuroradiol.* May
864 2011;32(5):798-808. doi:10.3174/ajnr.A2190
865 20.   Velat GJ, Chang SW, Abla AA, Albuquerque FC, McDougall CG, Spetzler RF.
866 Microsurgical management of glomus spinal arteriovenous malformations: pial resection
867 technique: Clinical article. *J Neurosurg Spine.* Jun 2012;16(6):523-31.
868 doi:10.3171/2012.3.SPINE11982
869 21.   Wilson DA, Abla AA, Uschold TD, McDougall CG, Albuquerque FC, Spetzler RF.
870 Multimodality treatment of conus medullaris arteriovenous malformations: 2 decades of
871 experience with combined endovascular and microsurgical treatments. *Neurosurgery.* Jul
872 2012;71(1):100-8. doi:10.1227/NEU.0b013e318256c042
873 22.   Bostrom A, Krings T, Hans FJ, Schramm J, Thron AK, Gilsbach JM. Spinal glomus-type
874 arteriovenous malformations: microsurgical treatment in 20 cases. *J Neurosurg Spine.* May
875 2009;10(5):423-9. doi:10.3171/2009.1.SPINE08355
876 23.   Kim LJ, Spetzler RF. Classification and surgical management of spinal arteriovenous
877 lesions: arteriovenous fistulae and arteriovenous malformations. *Neurosurgery.* Nov 2006;59(5
878 Suppl 3):S195-201; discussion S3-13. doi:10.1227/01.NEU.0000237335.82234.CE
879 24.   Sato K, Endo T, Niizuma K, et al. Concurrent dural and perimedullary arteriovenous
880 fistulas at the craniocervical junction: case series with special reference to angioarchitecture.
881 *Journal of neurosurgery.* 2013;118(2):451-459.
882 25.   Iampreechakul P, Lertbutsayanukul P, Siriwimonmas S. Cauda equina arteriovenous
883 fistula supplied by proximal radicular artery and concomitant sacral dural arteriovenous fistula:
884 A case report and literature review. *Surgical Neurology International.* 2021;12
885 26.   Dumont AS, Lanzino G, Sheehan JP. *Brain arteriovenous malformations and
886 arteriovenous fistulas.* Thieme; 2017.
887 27.   Niwa J, Matsumura S, Maeda Y, Ohoyama H. Transcondylar approach for dural
888 arteriovenous fistulas of the cervicomedullary junction. *Surgical neurology.* 1997;48(6):627-631.
889 28.   Llácer JL, Suay G, Piquer J, Vazquez V. Dural arteriovenous fistula at the foramen
890 magnum: report of a case and clinical-anatomical review. *Neurocirugia.* 2016;27(4):199-203.
891 29.   Zhou L-F, Chen L, Song D-L, Gu Y-X, Leng B. Tentorial dural arteriovenous fistulas.
892 *Surgical neurology.* 2007;67(5):472-481.
893 30.   Gross BA, Ropper AE, Du R. Cerebral dural arteriovenous fistulas and aneurysms.
894 *Neurosurgical focus.* 2012;32(5):E2.
895 31.   Strom RG, Botros JA, Refai D, et al. Cranial dural arteriovenous fistulae: asymptomatic
896 cortical venous drainage portends less aggressive clinical course. *Neurosurgery.* 2009;64(2):241-
897 248.
898 32.   Söderman M, Pavic L, Edner Gr, Holmin S, Andersson T. Natural history of dural
899 arteriovenous shunts. *Stroke.* 2008;39(6):1735-1739.
900 33.   Iampreechakul P, Wangtanaphat K, Wattanasen Y, Hangsapruek S, Lertbutsayanukul P,
901 Siriwimonmas S. Dural arteriovenous fistula of the craniocervical junction along the first
902 cervical nerve: A single-center experience and review of the literature. *Clinical Neurology and
903 Neurosurgery.* 2023/01/01/ 2023;224:107548. doi:https://doi.org/10.1016/j.clineuro.2022.107548

34.   Takai K, Endo T, Seki T, Inoue T, Koyanagi I, Mitsuhara T. Ischemic complications in the neurosurgical and endovascular treatments of craniocervical junction arteriovenous fistulas: a multicenter study. *Journal of Neurosurgery*. 2022;1(aop):1-10.

35.   Zhong W, Zhang J, Shen J, et al. Dural arteriovenous fistulas at the craniocervical junction: a series case report. *World Neurosurgery*. 2019;122:e700-e712.

36.   Hashimoto H, Iida J-i, Shin Y, Hironaka Y, Sakaki T. Spinal dural arteriovenous fistula with perimesencephalic subarachnoid haemorrhage. *Journal of clinical neuroscience*. 2000;7(1):64-66.

37.   Do HM, Jensen ME, Cloft HJ, Kallmes DF, Dion JE. Dural arteriovenous fistula of the cervical spine presenting with subarachnoid hemorrhage. *American Journal of Neuroradiology*. 1999;20(2):348-350.

38.   Aviv RI, Shad A, Tomlinson G, et al. Cervical dural arteriovenous fistulae manifesting as subarachnoid hemorrhage: report of two cases and literature review. *American Journal of Neuroradiology*. 2004;25(5):854-858.

39.   Chen G, Wang Q, Tian Y, et al. Dural arteriovenous fistulae at the craniocervical junction: the relation between clinical symptom and pattern of venous drainage. *Acta Neurochir Suppl*. 2011;110(Pt 2):99-104. doi:10.1007/978-3-7091-0356-2_18

40.   Kai Y, Hamada J-i, Morioka M, Yano S, Mizuno T, Kuratsu J-i. Arteriovenous fistulas at the cervicomedullary junction presenting with subarachnoid hemorrhage: six case reports with special reference to the angiographic pattern of venous drainage. *American journal of neuroradiology*. 2005;26(8):1949-1954.

41.   Spetzler RF, Martin NA. A proposed grading system for arteriovenous malformations. *J Neurosurg*. Oct 1986;65(4):476-83. doi:10.3171/jns.1986.65.4.0476

42.   Takai K, Komori T, Kurita H, Kawai K, Inoue T, Taniguchi M. Intradural radicular arteriovenous fistula that mimics dural arteriovenous fistula: report of three cases. *Neuroradiology*. Oct 2019;61(10):1203-1208. doi:10.1007/s00234-019-02275-0

43.   Guédon A, Saint-Maurice JP, Thépenier C, et al. Results of transvenous embolization of intracranial dural arteriovenous fistula: a consecutive series of 136 patients with 142 fistulas. *J Neurosurg*. May 28 2021:1-9. doi:10.3171/2020.10.Jns203604

44.   Salem MM, Srinivasan VM, Tonetti DA, et al. Microsurgical Obliteration of Craniocervical Junction Dural Arteriovenous Fistulas: Multicenter Experience. *Neurosurgery*. 2023;92(1)

45.   Fassett DR, Rammos SK, Patel P, Parikh H, Couldwell WT. Intracranial subarachnoid hemorrhage resulting from cervical spine dural arteriovenous fistulas: literature review and case presentation. *Neurosurg Focus*. Jan 2009;26(1):E4. doi:10.3171/foc.2009.26.1.E4

46.   Abiko M, Ikawa F, Ohbayashi N, Mitsuhara T, Ichinose N, Inagawa T. Endovascular treatment for dural arteriovenous fistula of the anterior condylar confluence involving the anterior condylar vein. A report of two cases. *Interv Neuroradiol*. Sep 30 2008;14(3):313-7. doi:10.1177/159101990801400312

47.   Agnoletto GJ, Fredrickson VL, Hollon TC, Couldwell WT. Far Lateral Craniotomy for Obliteration of High-Risk Craniocervical Junction Arteriovenous Fistula. *Neurol India*. Nov-Dec 2021;69(6):1554-1556. doi:10.4103/0028-3886.333526

48.   Alshekhlee A, Edgell RC, Kale SP, Kitchener J, Vora N. Endovascular Therapy of a Craniocervical Pial AVF Fed by the Anterior Spinal Artery. *Journal of Neuroimaging*. 2013;23(1):102-104. doi:https://doi.org/10.1111/j.1552-6569.2010.00569.x

949 49.   Ansari SA, Lassig JP, Nicol E, Thompson BG, Gemmete JJ, Gandhi D. Transarterial
950 embolization of a cervical dural arteriovenous fistula. Presenting with subarachnoid hemorrhage.
951 *Interv Neuroradiol*. Dec 15 2006;12(4):313-8. doi:10.1177/159101990601200404
952 50.   Arai N, Akiyama T, Yoshida K. The Coexistence of Extradural Arteriovenous Fistula and
953 Soft Tissue Arteriovenous Malformation Within the Same Metamere. *World Neurosurg*. Feb
954 2017;98:877.e1-877.e7. doi:10.1016/j.wneu.2016.11.076
955 51.   Asakawa H, Yanaka K, Fujita K, Marushima A, Anno I, Nose T. Intracranial dural
956 arteriovenous fistula showing diffuse MR enhancement of the spinal cord: case report and review
957 of the literature. *Surg Neurol*. Sep-Oct 2002;58(3-4):251-7. doi:10.1016/s0090-3019(02)00861-3
958 52.   Beynon C, Herweh C, Rohde S, Unterberg AW, Sakowitz OW. Intraoperative
959 indocyanine green angiography for microsurgical treatment of a craniocervical dural
960 arteriovenous fistula. *Clin Neurol Neurosurg*. Jul 2012;114(6):696-8.
961 doi:10.1016/j.clineuro.2011.11.022
962 53.   Chan N. Hypoglossal dural arteriovenous fistula: a rare cause of unilateral hypoglossal
963 nerve palsy. *BJR Case Rep*. 2017;3(3):20160144. doi:10.1259/bjrcr.20160144
964 54.   Choi HS, Kim DI, Kim BM, Kim DJ, Ahn SS. Endovascular treatment of dural
965 arteriovenous fistula involving marginal sinus with emphasis on the routes of transvenous
966 embolization. *Neuroradiology*. Feb 2012;54(2):163-9. doi:10.1007/s00234-011-0852-4
967 55.   Do HM, Jensen ME, Cloft HJ, Kallmes DF, Dion JE. Dural arteriovenous fistula of the
968 cervical spine presenting with subarachnoid hemorrhage. *AJNR Am J Neuroradiol*. Feb
969 1999;20(2):348-50.
970 56.   Doniselli FM, Paolucci A, Conte G, Rampini P, Arrichiello A, Triulzi FM. Glue
971 embolization of a pial arteriovenous fistula of the spinal artery. *Acta Biomed*. Sep 23
972 2020;91(10-s):e2020004. doi:10.23750/abm.v91i10-S.10282
973 57.   Enokizono M, Sato N, Morikawa M, et al. "Black butterfly" sign on T2*-weighted and
974 susceptibility-weighted imaging: A novel finding of chronic venous congestion of the brain stem
975 and spinal cord associated with dural arteriovenous fistulas. *J Neurol Sci*. Aug 15 2017;379:64-
976 68. doi:10.1016/j.jns.2017.05.066
977 58.   Firsching R, Kohl J, Skalej M, Beuing O. Resolution of Brainstem Edema after
978 Neurosurgical Occlusion of Dural Arteriovenous Fistulas of the Craniocervical Junction: Report
979 of Three Cases and Review. *J Neurol Surg A Cent Eur Neurosurg*. Jan 2020;81(1):80-85.
980 doi:10.1055/s-0039-1688560
981 59.   Gadot R, Gopakumar S, Wagner K, et al. Foramen Magnum Dural Arteriovenous Fistula
982 Presenting With Thoracic Myelopathy: Technical Case Report With 2-Dimensional Operative
983 Video. *Oper Neurosurg (Hagerstown)*. Jun 15 2021;21(1):E55-e59. doi:10.1093/ons/opab077
984 60.   Gilard V, Curey S, Tollard E, Proust F. Coincidental vascular anomalies at the foramen
985 magnum: dural arteriovenous fistula and high flow aneurysm on perimedullary fistula.
986 *Neurochirurgie*. Dec 2013;59(6):210-3. doi:10.1016/j.neuchi.2013.06.003
987 61.   Hasegawa H, Bitoh S, Katoh A, Tamura K. Bilateral vertebral arteriovenous fistulas and
988 atlantoaxial dislocation associated with neurofibromatosis--case report. *Neurol Med Chir*
989 *(Tokyo)*. Jan 1989;29(1):55-9. doi:10.2176/nmc.29.55
990 62.   Hashimoto Y, Kin S, Haraguchi K, Niwa J. Pitfalls in the preoperative evaluation of
991 subarachnoid hemorrhage without digital subtraction angiography: report on 2 cases. *Surg
992 Neurol*. Sep 2007;68(3):344-8. doi:10.1016/j.surneu.2006.10.057
993 63.   Hayashi N, Tomura N, Okada H, et al. Usefulness of preoperative cone beam computed
994 tomography and intraoperative digital subtraction angiography for dural arteriovenous fistula at

craniocervical junction: Technical case report. *Surg Neurol Int*. 2019;10:5. doi:10.4103/sni.sni_439_17

64.   Horiuchi R, Kanemaru K, Yoshioka H, et al. Endoscope-Integrated Fluorescence Video Angiography for the Surgery of Ventrally Located Perimedullary Arteriovenous Fistula at Craniocervical Junction. *World Neurosurg*. May 2020;137:126-129. doi:10.1016/j.wneu.2020.01.207

65.   Hurst RW, Bagley LJ, Scanlon M, Flamm ES. Dural arteriovenous fistulas of the craniocervical junction. *Skull Base Surg*. 1999;9(1):1-7. doi:10.1055/s-2008-1058166

66.   Inamasu J, Tanaka R, Nakahara I, Hirose Y. Dural arteriovenous fistula of the craniocervical junction manifesting as cerebellar haemorrhage. *Neuroradiol J*. Oct 2016;29(5):356-60. doi:10.1177/1971400916665374

67.   Inci S, Bertan V, Cila A. Angiographically occult epidural arteriovenous fistula of the craniocervical junction. *Surg Neurol*. Mar 2002;57(3):167-73; discussion 173. doi:10.1016/s0090-3019(02)00631-6

68.   Jeon JP, Cho YD, Kim CH, Han MH. Complex spinal arteriovenous fistula of the craniocervical junction with pial and dural shunts combined with contralateral dural arteriovenous fistula. *Interv Neuroradiol*. Dec 2015;21(6):733-7. doi:10.1177/1591019915609128

69.   Jiang P, Lv X, Wu Z, Li Y. Dural arteriovenous fistula of crianiocervical junction: Four case reports. *Neurol India*. Jan-Feb 2012;60(1):94-5. doi:10.4103/0028-3886.93612

70.   Kanemaru K, Yoshioka H, Hashimoto K, et al. Efficacy of Intraarterial Fluorescence Video Angiography in Surgery for Dural and Perimedullary Arteriovenous Fistula at Craniocervical Junction. *World Neurosurg*. Jun 2019;126:e573-e579. doi:10.1016/j.wneu.2019.02.097

71.   Kasliwal MK, Moftakhar R, O'Toole JE, Lopes DK. High cervical spinal subdural hemorrhage as a harbinger of craniocervical arteriovenous fistula: an unusual clinical presentation. *Spine J*. May 1 2015;15(5):e13-7. doi:10.1016/j.spinee.2015.02.035

72.   Kattner KA, Roth TC, Giannotta SL. Cranial base approaches for the surgical treatment of aggressive posterior fossa dural arteriovenous fistulae with leptomeningeal drainage: report of four technical cases. *Neurosurgery*. May 2002;50(5):1156-60; discussion 1160-1. doi:10.1097/00006123-200205000-00042

73.   Kattner KA, Roth TC, Nardone EM, Giannotta SL. The treatment of complex dural arteriovenous fistulae through cranial base techniques. *Neurol India*. Sep 2004;52(3):325-31.

74.   Kawasaki T, Fukuda H, Kurosaki Y, Handa A, Chin M, Yamagata S. Acute Compressive Myelopathy Caused by Spinal Subarachnoid Hemorrhage: A Combined Effect of Asymptomatic Cervical Spondylosis. *World Neurosurg*. Nov 2016;95:619.e1-619.e4. doi:10.1016/j.wneu.2016.08.031

75.   Kida Y. Radiosurgery for dural arteriovenous fistula. *Prog Neurol Surg*. 2009;22:38-44. doi:10.1159/000163381

76.   Kidd J. Traumatic vertebral artery arteriovenous fistula. *Journal for Vascular Ultrasound*. 2015;39(1):21-24.

77.   Kikkawa Y, Nakamizo A, Yamashita K, Amano T, Kurogi A, Sasaki T. Preoperative evaluation and surgical strategies for craniocervical junction dural arteriovenous fistula with multiple feeders: case report and review of the literature. *Fukuoka Igaku Zasshi*. Sep 2013;104(9):299-308.

1040   78.   Kiyosue H, Okahara M, Sagara Y, et al. Dural arteriovenous fistula involving the
1041   posterior condylar canal. *AJNR Am J Neuroradiol*. Sep 2007;28(8):1599-601.
1042   doi:10.3174/ajnr.A0606
1043   79.   Kleeberg J, Maeder-Ingvar M, Maeder P. Progressive cervical myelopathy due to dural
1044   craniocervical fistula. *Eur Neurol*. 2010;63(6):374. doi:10.1159/000292430
1045   80.   Krishnan D, Viswanathan S, Rose N, Benjamin HSN, Ong AM, Hiew FL. Clinical
1046   heterogeneity of low flow spinal arteriovenous fistulas; a case series. *BMC Neurol*. Sep 21
1047   2021;21(1):366. doi:10.1186/s12883-021-02394-3
1048   81.   Kulwin C, Bohnstedt BN, Scott JA, Cohen-Gadol A. Dural arteriovenous fistulas
1049   presenting with brainstem dysfunction: diagnosis and surgical treatment. *Neurosurg Focus*. May
1050   2012;32(5):E10. doi:10.3171/2012.2.Focus1217
1051   82.   Kuwayama N, Kubo M, Nishijima M, Horie Y, Endo S, Takaku A. Treatment of
1052   intracranial (dural) arteriovenous fistulas in unusual locations. *Interv Neuroradiol*. Nov 1999;5
1053   Suppl 1:115-20. doi:10.1177/15910199990050s121
1054   83.   Lam SKS, Chu SL, Yuen SC, Yam KY. Far Lateral Approach for Disconnection of
1055   Craniocervical Junction Dural Arteriovenous Fistula Presented with Myelopathy and
1056   Hydrocephalus. *J Neurol Surg B Skull Base*. Feb 2021;82(Suppl 1):S45-s47. doi:10.1055/s-0040-
1057   1714402
1058   84.   Lang MJ, Atallah E, Tjoumakaris S, Rosenwasser RH, Jabbour P. Remote Thoracic
1059   Myelopathy From a Spinal Dural Arteriovenous Fistula at the Craniocervical Junction: Case
1060   Report and Review of Literature. *World Neurosurg*. Dec 2017;108:992.e1-992.e4.
1061   doi:10.1016/j.wneu.2017.08.158
1062   85.   Lin I-C, Wu H-C, Wu C-H, Lin W-C, Lieu A-S. Craniocervical junction spinal dural
1063   arteriovenous fistula presenting with progressive myelopathy and sudden deterioration.
1064   *Formosan Journal of Surgery*. 2017;50(6):223.
1065   86.   Liu X, Ogata A, Masuoka J, et al. Dural arteriovenous fistula manifesting as pontine
1066   hemorrhage at the craniocervical junction. *Acta Neurochir (Wien)*. May 2017;159(5):831-834.
1067   doi:10.1007/s00701-017-3135-y
1068   87.   Liu M, Tian DS. The "tigroid" pattern of medullary lesion in craniocervical dural
1069   arteriovenous fistula: A neglected radiological finding. *J Neuroradiol*. Jun 2022;49(4):352-353.
1070   doi:10.1016/j.neurad.2021.12.004
1071   88.   Lv X, Yang X, Li Y, Jiang C, Wu Z. Dural arteriovenous fistula with spinal
1072   perimedullary venous drainage. *Neurol India*. Nov-Dec 2011;59(6):899-902. doi:10.4103/0028-
1073   3886.91374
1074   89.   Mascalchi M, Scazzeri F, Prosetti D, Ferrito G, Salvi F, Quilici N. Dural arteriovenous
1075   fistula at the craniocervical junction with perimedullary venous drainage. *AJNR Am J
1076   Neuroradiol*. Jun-Jul 1996;17(6):1137-41.
1077   90.   Maus V, Söderman M, Rodesch G, Kabbasch C, Mpotsaris A. Endovascular treatment of
1078   posterior condylar canal dural arteriovenous fistula. *J Neurointerv Surg*. Feb 2017;9(2):e7.
1079   doi:10.1136/neurintsurg-2016-012384.rep
1080   91.   Naylor RM, Topinka B, Rinaldo L, et al. Progressive Myelopathy From a Craniocervical
1081   Junction Dural Arteriovenous Fistula. *Stroke*. Jun 2021;52(6):e278-e281.
1082   doi:10.1161/strokeaha.120.032552
1083   92.   Oishi H, Okuda O, Arai H, Maehara T, Iizuka Y. Successful surgical treatment of a dural
1084   arteriovenous fistula at the craniocervical junction with reference to pre- and postoperative MRI.
1085   *Neuroradiology*. Jun 1999;41(6):463-7. doi:10.1007/s002340050785

93.   Okamoto T, Nanto M, Hasegawa Y, et al. Early rebleeding of a foramen magnum dural arteriovenous fistula: A case report and review of the literature. *Radiol Case Rep.* Nov 2021;16(11):3499-3503. doi:10.1016/j.radcr.2021.08.038

94.   Oshita J, Yamaguchi S, Ohba S, Kurisu K. Mirror-image spinal dural arteriovenous fistulas at the craniocervical junction: case report and review of the literature. *Neurosurgery.* Nov 2011;69(5):E1166-71. doi:10.1227/NEU.0b013e318223bab5

95.   Peltier J, Baroncini M, Thines L, Lacour A, Leclerc X, Lejeune JP. Subacute involvement of the medulla oblongata and occipital neuralgia revealing an intracranial dural arteriovenous fistula of the craniocervical junction. *Neurol India.* Mar-Apr 2011;59(2):285-8. doi:10.4103/0028-3886.79153

96.   Pop R, Manisor M, Aloraini Z, et al. Foramen magnum dural arteriovenous fistula presenting with epilepsy. *Interv Neuroradiol.* Dec 2015;21(6):724-7. doi:10.1177/1591019915609783

97.   Salamon E, Patsalides A, Gobin YP, Santillan A, Fink ME. Dural arteriovenous fistula at the craniocervical junction mimicking acute brainstem and spinal cord infarction. *JAMA Neurol.* Jun 2013;70(6):796-7. doi:10.1001/jamaneurol.2013.1946

98.   Sasada S, Hiramatsu M, Kusumegi A, et al. Arteriovenous Fistula at the Craniocervical Junction Found After Cervical Laminoplasty for Ossification of the Posterior Longitudinal Ligament. *Neurospine.* Dec 2020;17(4):947-953. doi:10.14245/ns.2040200.100

99.   Sasaki K, Inoue T, Inoue T, et al. Intractable Hiccups as the Primary Symptom of a Perimedullary Arteriovenous Fistula at the Craniocervical Junction. *World Neurosurg.* Sep 2020;141:64-68. doi:10.1016/j.wneu.2020.06.013

100.   Sato H, Wada H, Noro S, Saga T, Kamada K. Subarachnoid Hemorrhage with Concurrent Dural and Perimedullary Arteriovenous Fistulas at Craniocervical Junction: Case Report and Literature Review. *World Neurosurg.* Jul 2019;127:331-334. doi:10.1016/j.wneu.2019.02.079

101.   Shinoyama M, Endo T, Takahash T, et al. Long-term outcome of cervical and thoracolumbar dural arteriovenous fistulas with emphasis on sensory disturbance and neuropathic pain. *World Neurosurg.* Apr 2010;73(4):401-8. doi:10.1016/j.wneu.2010.01.003

102.   Sorenson TJ, De Maria L, Rangel-Castilla L, Lanzino G. Surgical treatment of previously embolized craniocervical junction dural arteriovenous fistula. *Neurosurg Focus.* Apr 1 2019;46(Suppl_2):V2. doi:10.3171/2019.2.FocusVid.18639

103.   Suda S, Katsura K, Okubo S, et al. A case of dural arteriovenous fistulas at the craniocervical junction presenting with occipital/neck pain associated with sleep. *Intern Med.* 2012;51(8):925-8. doi:10.2169/internalmedicine.51.6607

104.   Sun L, Ren J, Zhang H. Application of the selective indocyanine green videoangiography in microsurgical treatment of a craniocervical junction dural arteriovenous fistula. *Neurosurg Focus.* Apr 1 2019;46(Suppl_2):V5. doi:10.3171/2019.2.FocusVid.18681

105.   Sutiono AB, Banjarnahor JD. A case involving a giant aberrant craniocervical arteriovenous malformation. *Surg Neurol Int.* 2019;10:99. doi:10.25259/sni-161-2019

106.   Takahashi H, Ueshima T, Goto D, et al. Acute Tetraparesis with Respiratory Failure after Steroid Administration in a Patient with a Dural Arteriovenous Fistula at the Craniocervical Junction. *Intern Med.* Feb 15 2018;57(4):591-594. doi:10.2169/internalmedicine.9115-17

107.   Takamatsu S, Suzuki K, Murakami Y, Nomura K, Yamamoto J, Nishizawa S. Usefulness of arterial spin labeling in the evaluation for dural arteriovenous fistula of the craniocervical junction. *Radiol Case Rep.* Jul 2021;16(7):1655-1659. doi:10.1016/j.radcr.2021.04.006

1132   108.   Tong X, Jiang Z, Ye M, Zhang H. Craniocervical junction dural arteriovenous fistula
1133   with rare fistulous site. *J Neurosurg Sci*. Aug 2021;65(4):456-457. doi:10.23736/s0390-
1134   5616.20.05032-8
1135   109.   Trop I, Roy D, Raymond J, Roux A, Bourgouin P, Lesage J. Craniocervical dural fistula
1136   associated with cervical myelopathy: angiographic demonstration of normal venous drainage of
1137   the thoracolumbar cord does not rule out diagnosis. *AJNR Am J Neuroradiol*. Mar
1138   1998;19(3):583-6.
1139   110.   Willinsky R, TerBrugge K, Lasjaunias P, Montanera W. The variable presentations of
1140   craniocervical and cervical dural arteriovenous malformations. *Surg Neurol*. Aug
1141   1990;34(2):118-23. doi:10.1016/0090-3019(90)90107-z
1142   111.   Wu Q, Wang HD, Shin YS, Zhang X. Brainstem Congestion due to Dural Ateriovenous
1143   Fistula at the Craniocervical Junction. *J Korean Neurosurg Soc*. Mar 2014;55(3):152-5.
1144   doi:10.3340/jkns.2014.55.3.152
1145   112.   Yamashita T, Takehara S, Miyazaki K, Kitahama Y, Namba H. Enhanced MR
1146   angiography for depiction of spinal dural arteriovenous fistula in the craniocervical junction. *J
1147   Neuroradiol*. Jul 2011;38(3):196-8. doi:10.1016/j.neurad.2010.08.003
1148   113.   Yoo DH, Cho YD, Boonchai T, et al. Endovascular treatment of medullary bridging vein-
1149   draining dural arteriovenous fistulas: foramen magnum vs. craniocervical junction lesions.
1150   *Neuroradiology*. Feb 2022;64(2):333-342. doi:10.1007/s00234-021-02790-z
1151   114.   Yoshida K, Sato S, Inoue T, et al. Transvenous embolization for craniocervical junction
1152   epidural arteriovenous fistula with a pial feeder aneurysm. *Interv Neuroradiol*. Apr
1153   2020;26(2):170-177. doi:10.1177/1591019919874571

1154

1155

1156

1157

1158

1159

1160

1161

1162

1163   **Figure Legend**

1164   **Figure 1**. PRISMA diagram detailing study selection process utilized during systematic review.

1165

1166
1167

Brown, Nolan (Medical Student)
Deleted: Figure 2. Example of symptomatic presentation and radiographic diagnosis of CCJ DAVF in a 59-year-old female with no history of traumatic injury who presented with slowly progressive spastic tetraparesis, bulbar symptoms, dysphagia, dysarthria. MRI is recommended for patients with myelopathy of the upper cervical cord. (A) Sagittal FLAIR demonstrating high brainstem signal due to tortuous vessels and vasogenic edema. (B) Axial T2 MRI showing increased signal intensity with tortuous vessels in the subarachnoid space and resulting vasogenic edema. (C) Sagittal T1 MRI demonstration low brainstem signal intensity resulting from vasogenic edema. (D) Sagittal T2 MRI with high signal intensity from brainstem down to spinal cord and tortuous veins in subarachnoid space. Edematous change resulting from enlarged and tortuous subarachnoid vasculature is highly suggestive of DAVF. In order to confirm the specific diagnosis, selective digital subtraction angiography (DSA) should be performed. (E) 3D rotational DSA shows DAVF with engorgement of veins surrounding spinal cord and brainstem; at this point percutaneous embolization can be considered and its use will vary on a case-by-case basis. Ultimately, this presentation is consistent with acquired DAVF located at the CCJ, a rare entity especially in the absence of any history of prior trauma. This case was made available by radiopaedia.org.

Appendix 3: An Example of a Response to Reviewers Document

Reviewer 1

"The authors, through an institutional retrospective analysis of diabetes outcomes, find that less insulin control is associated with higher short-term readmission rates. This finding is exciting; however, as the patients are from a heterogenous age profile and demographic profile, these confounding factors could have influenced outcomes."

Author response:

We thank the reviewer for taking the time to read our manuscript and for providing helpful feedback. In order to control for demographic and clinical factors that may influence outcomes, we performed a multivariate analysis (Table 3). Taking these additional factors into account, poor glucose control still significantly and independently predicted short-term readmission.

Changes to Text: Added Table 3.

"The 'blind spots' in diabetes control also need a mention along with how diabetes control can be modified to assess outcomes."

Author response:

We thank the reviewer for their insightful comment and important note on the specificity of the diabetic control measurement system. We have added additional discussion on the applicability of this system to the manuscript. Further, given the lack of available literature on diabetic control-specific indices, we have added an additional note to the limitations section indicating this may be a future direction for research.

Changes to text:

"Importantly, the diabetic control scale is one of many indices that have proven useful in predicting short-term readmission. Despite its widespread and generalized use, the diabetes control scale has been found to be particularly relevant for these patient cohorts." (Lines 189–192)

"Moreover, this diabetes control scale may be of value when considering predictive metrics for short-term readmission outcomes. As a result, future research may look to form diabetic control-specific indices." (Lines 211–214)

Reviewer 2

"The authors retrospectively reviewed the records of all patients with uncontrolled diabetes undergoing treatment by a medical provider at one department. They retrieved 263 cases. As a result, they found that a patient's insulin control was independently and significantly associated

with short-term readmission. The paper was prepared in a straightforward manner but it has no new contribution to present literature."

Author response:

We thank the reviewer for their feedback and for taking the time to help us improve our work. We hope that primary care providers and endocrinologists will find our results useful in their patient counseling efforts and as they coordinate care for patients suffering from severe diabetes.

Furthermore, we hope that by addressing the comments from Reviewers 1 and 2, our manuscript is now suitable for publication in the peer-reviewed literature.

<u>Reviewer 3</u>

"1. How many patients required short-acting insulin in addition to long-acting insulin?"

Author response:

We appreciate the reviewer taking note of this important data point and have added an additional statement to the results indicating how many patients required long-acting insulin.

Changes to text:

"137 patients had short-acting insulin for glucose control (52.1) and 91 patients (34.6) required a long-acting insulin." (Lines 95–98)

"2. What was the reason for readmission? Was it always infection or wound complications?"

Author response:

We thank the reviewer for their helpful comment and agree that this information is of critical importance. We added a discussion of this information to the results section.

Changes to text:

"Regarding the reason for readmission, all patients were readmitted for infection wound complication. Notably, no patients were readmitted for the hyperosmolar syndrome." (Lines 114–115)

Appendix 4:
An Example of a United States Patent

(12) **United States Patent**
Long, III

(10) **Patent No.:**   **US 6,360,693 B1**
(45) **Date of Patent:**   **Mar. 26, 2002**

(54) **ANIMAL TOY**

(76) Inventor: **Ross Eugene Long, III**, 4732 Reinhardt Dr., Oakland, CA (US) 94619

(*) Notice: Subject to any disclaimer, the term of this patent is extended or adjusted under 35 U.S.C. 154(b) by 0 days.

(21) Appl. No.: **09/454,229**

(22) Filed: **Dec. 2, 1999**

(51) **Int. Cl.**[7] **A01K 29/00**
(52) **U.S. Cl.** **119/707**
(58) **Field of Search** 119/702, 707, 119/709, 710, 711, 467, 468, 256, 268

(56)   **References Cited**

U.S. PATENT DOCUMENTS

1,006,182	A	*	10/1911	Cousin	119/710
1,022,113	A	*	4/1912	Smith	119/710
3,830,202	A	*	8/1974	Garrison	119/710
4,202,922	A	*	5/1980	Osment	428/18
5,018,480	A	*	5/1991	Goldman et al.	119/26
RE34,352	E	*	8/1993	Markham et al.	119/710
5,752,463	A	*	5/1998	Jenkins	119/57.8
5,819,687	A	*	10/1998	Lister	119/52.1

* cited by examiner

Primary Examiner—Thomas Price

(57)   **ABSTRACT**

An apparatus for use as a toy by an animal, for example a dog, to either fetch carry or chew includes a main section with at least one protrusion extending therefrom that resembles a branch in appearance. The toy is formed of any of a number of materials including rubber, plastic, or wood including wood composites and is solid. It is either rigid or flexible. A flavoring (scent) is added, if desired. The toy is adapted to float by including a material therein that is lighter than water or it is adapted to glow in the dark, as desired, by the addition of a fluorescent material that is either included in the material from which the toy is made or the flourescent material is applied thereto as a coating. The toy may be segmented (i.e., notched) so as to break off into smaller segments, as is useful for smaller animals or, alternatively, to extend the life of the toy. Various textured surfaces including camouflage colorings are anticipated as are straight or curved main sections. The toy may be formed of any desired material, as described, so as to be edible by the animal.

20 Claims, 3 Drawing Sheets

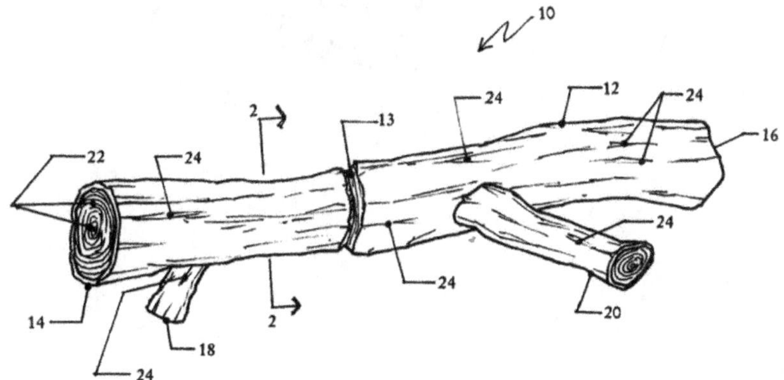

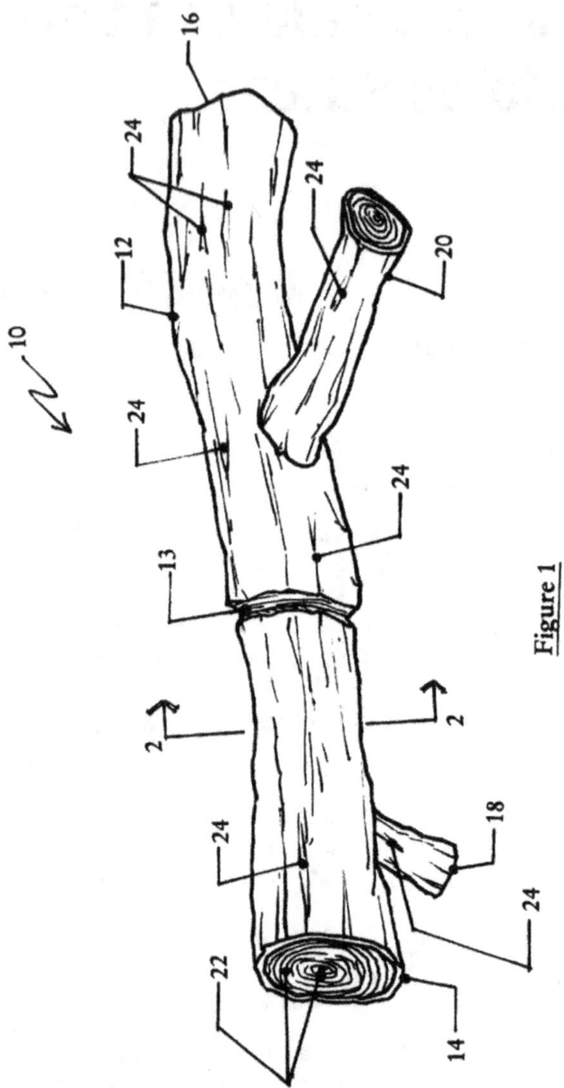

Figure 1

U.S. Patent   Mar. 26, 2002   Sheet 2 of 3   US 6,360,693 B1

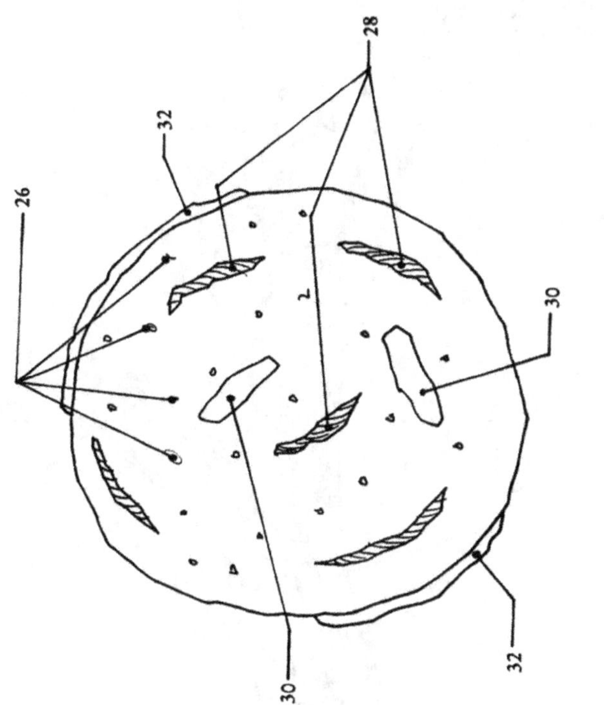

U.S. Patent   Mar. 26, 2002   Sheet 3 of 3   **US 6,360,693 B1**

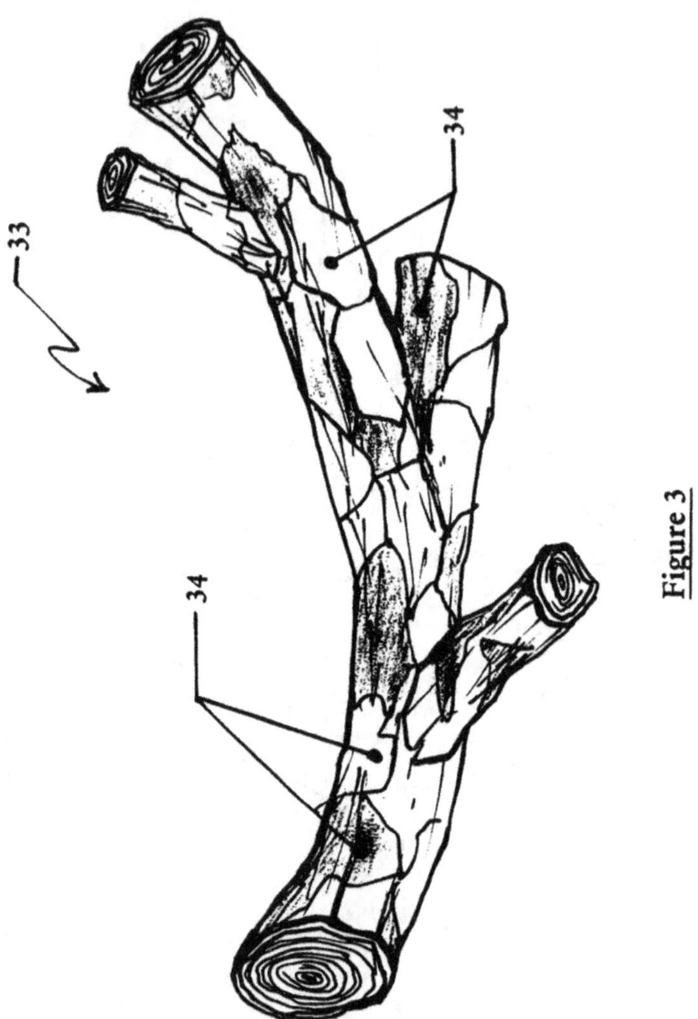

US 6,360,693 B1

<table>
<tr><td>

1

ANIMAL TOY

BACKGROUND OF THE INVENTION

1. Field of the Invention

The present invention, in general relates to animal toys and, more particularly, to devices that a dog can chew and carry in its mouth.

Dog chew toys are well known and include a wide variety of devices, some of which rapidly disintegrate—as is well known to most dog owners.

Other dog chew toys are sometimes used in fetching training exercises or simply for play but they may be difficult for the dog to pick up off of the ground. If tossed onto a body of water, they may sink. Furthermore, while a dog may see the toy at night or in dim light, the owner is unable to do so and therefore the toy cannot be used in dim light.

Other variations, such as it being edible or chewable (to relieve the natural tendency dogs have to chew) are also desirable features to incorporate in any dog chew toy design.

It is a natural tendency for dogs to chew and they often make inappropriate selections as to what they will chew. A scented or flavored animal toy that encourages a dog to chew, and possibly to consume it, would be useful.

When training dogs, especially hunting dogs, to fetch or when deciding which dog is especially good for the scent discrimination purpose, it is necessary to asses their ability to detect objects based solely on scent. Therefore an animal toy that is camouflaged would be useful in training and determining a dog's ability to locate hard to find objects based solely on scent.

Accordingly there exists today a need for an animal toy that floats, is easy to pick up off of the ground, can be seen in dim light, is made from a variety of possible materials, and which dogs may chew.

Clearly, such an apparatus would be a useful and desirable device.

2. Description of Prior Art

Dog toys are, in general, known. For example, the following patents describe various types of these devices:

U.S. Pat. No. 3,830,202 to Garrison, Aug. 20, 1974;

U.S. Pat. No. 4,133,296 to Smith, Jan. 9, 1979;

U.S. Pat. No. 4,557,219 to Edwards, Dec. 10, 1985;

U.S. Pat. No. 4,919,083 to Axelrod, Apr. 24, 1990;

U.S. Pat. No. 5,263,436 to Axelrod, Nov. 23, 1993;

U.S. Pat. No. 5,269,256 to Viola, Dec. 14, 1993;

U.S. Pat. No. 5,415,132 to Meyer, May 16, 1995;

U.S. Pat. No. 5,711,254 to O'Rourke, Jan. 27, 1998;

U.S. Pat. No. 5,904,118 to Markham, May 18, 1999;

and the following design patents:

U.S. Des. Pat. No. 319,605 to Jenks, Sep. 3, 1991;

U.S. Des. Pat. No. 327,962 to O'Rourke, Jul. 14, 1992;

U.S. Des. Pat. No. 329,310 to O'Rourke, Sep. 8, 1992;

U.S. Des. Pat. No. 330,614 to O'Rourke, Oct. 27, 1992;

U.S. Des. Pat. No. 330,921 to LaMagna, Nov. 10, 1992;

U.S. Des. Pat. No. 343,930 to Garcia, Feb. 1, 1994;

U.S. Des. Pat. No. 348,959 to Lawson, Jul. 19, 1994;

U.S. Des. Pat. No. 356,879 to O'Rourke, Mar. 28, 1995; and

U.S. Des. Pat. No. 368,932 to Mussalo, Apr. 16, 1996;

While the structural arrangements of the above described devices, at first appearance, have similarities with the

</td><td>

2

present invention, they differ in material respects. These differences, which will be described in more detail hereinafter, are essential for the effective use of the invention and which admit of the advantages that are not available with the prior devices.

OBJECTS AND SUMMARY OF THE INVENTION

It is an object of the present invention to provide an animal toy that a dog may carry in its mouth.

It is also an important object of the invention to provide an animal toy that is easy for a dog to pick up off of the ground.

Another object of the invention is to provide an animal toy that can float.

Still another object of the invention is to provide an animal toy that is visible in the dark.

Still yet another object of the invention is to provide an animal toy that glows in the dark.

Yet another important object of the invention is to provide an animal toy that can be used to teach a dog to fetch on land.

Still yet another important object of the invention is to provide an animal toy that can be used to teach a dog to fetch from the water.

It is a useful object of the invention is to provide an animal toy that is made of a material that a dog may chew.

It is a further useful object of the invention is to provide an animal toy that is made from wood.

It is a still further useful object of the invention is to provide an animal toy that is made from cellulose.

It is another useful object of the invention is to provide an animal toy that includes a cellulose and a binding agent or a resin.

It is a beneficial object of the invention is to provide an animal toy that includes a flavor added thereto.

It is a further beneficial object of the invention is to provide an animal toy that is chewable.

It is a still other beneficial object of the invention is to provide an animal toy that is formed of any desired color.

It is a useful and beneficial object of the invention is to provide an animal toy that resembles in appearance a branch segment.

It is another useful and beneficial object of the invention is to provide an animal toy that includes a textured surface that resembles a bark from a tree.

It is one further useful and beneficial object of the invention is to provide an animal toy that is rigid.

It is still one further useful and beneficial object of the invention is to provide an animal toy that is flexible.

It is still one further useful and beneficial object of the invention is to provide an animal toy that includes at least one break-off segment.

It is still one additional further useful and beneficial object of the invention is to provide an animal toy that includes a camouflage covering or texture surface.

Briefly, an animal toy that is constructed in accordance with the principles of the present invention has a straight or curved segment with at least one protrusion extending therefrom that resembles in appearance a branch. The animal toy is of any size and may be either flexible or rigid, floatable, chewable, edible, and the like depending upon the material that it is made from, including plastic, rubber, wood, and wood composites. A flavoring (or scent) may be

</td></tr>
</table>

US 6,360,693 B1

<table>
<tr><td>

3

added to the animal toy to encourage a dog to chew and possibly to consume the animal toy, depending upon what it is made from. Break-away notches are provided, as desired, to permit the animal toy to be broken into smaller segments. A glow in the dark material may be included with the animal toy to make it easier to use in the dark. Conversely, it may include a camouflage covering.

BRIEF DESCRIPTION OF THE DRAWINGS

FIG. 1 is a view in perspective of an animal toy.

FIG. 2 is an enlarged cross sectional view taken on the line 2—2 in FIG. 1 of a possible modified embodiment.

FIG. 3 is a view in perspective of an alternate camouflage embodiment of an animal toy illustrating a more curved shape.

DETAILED DESCRIPTION OF THE INVENTION

Referring to FIG. 1 is shown, an animal toy, identified in general by the reference numeral **10**.

The animal toy **10** is formed of any of a variety of materials depending upon the characteristics that are desired, including plastic, rubber, wood, and wood composites to name a few.

The animal toy **10** includes a main section **12** with a notch **13** disposed around its perimeter intermediate a first end **14** and a second end **16**.

The notch **13** creates a weak area along the main section **12** where, by applying a pressure, the animal toy **10** may be broken into two pieces. This is useful to extend its life or when it is to be used with smaller types of dogs.

Of course, if additional notches (not shown) are used, the animal toy **10** may be broken into more than two pieces.

Attached to and extending away from the main section **12** is a first protrusion **18** and a second protrusion **20**. At least one, namely the first protrusion **18**, is required for use with the animal toy **10** in order to realize its advantages. Accordingly, when the animal toy **10** is broken into two (or more) pieces, it is desirable that each piece include at least one of the first or second protrusions **18**, **20**.

The use of at least one of the first or second protrusions **18**, **20** ensures that the animal toy **10** will provide an irregular and somewhat raised portion above a ground surface upon which the animal toy **10** is placed (or lands if it is thrown). The irregular and raised portions make it easier for a dog (not shown) to pick up and carry the animal toy in its mouth.

The first end **14** of the animal toy **10** includes a plurality of rings **22** that resemble those of a stick or branch. To further the illusion of being a stick or a branch, a simulated textured bark **24** is disposed along the longitudinal length of the animal toy **10**.

Referring now also to FIG. **2**, is shown a variety of possible modifications to the animal toy **10**. The animal toy **10** is formed of a plurality of cellulose (wood) fibers **26** that are held together in the desired shape by pressing them tightly together, in a manner similar to that which particle board, a building material (not shown), is formed in which the natural resins act as a binding agent under pressure.

Any preferred type of a wood may be used. The fibers **26** are of any preferred size and include small particles to larger chips.

If it is desirable to encourage the dog to chew on the animal toy **10**, a layering of a flavoring **28** is added throughout the animal toy **10**, as desired.

</td><td>

4

The flavoring **28** provides both a flavor and a scent that encourages the dog to chew or play with the animal toy **10**.

Depending upon the material used to form the animal toy **10** it may be desirable that the dog actually consume (eat) the animal toy **10**. For example, it may contain various types of dietary fibers beneficial to the dogs digestive system. These fibers may also be added to the animal toy **10** as a separate ingredient when it is formed or they may be a natural by-product arising from the materials, such as wood, that are alternatively used to form the animal toy **10**.

Some materials have a specific gravity that is less than that of water and so the animal toy **10** will naturally float. If that is not the case and it is desirable that the animal toy **10** should float, then a plurality of pockets **30** are provided when the animal toy **10** is formed. The pockets **30** contain any preferred material that includes a specific gravity that is less than that of water (i.e., that is lighter than water).

Accordingly, the animal toy **10** does not contain any voids.

A fluorescent coating **32** is applied where desired to the surface of the animal toy **10** (or mixed into the forming material) so that it may glow in the dark. This permits use of the animal toy **10** under low light conditions.

Of course, the animal toy **10** may be formed of any desired color. The simulated textured bark **24** may be of any depth or color or pattern, as desired.

However, a modified animal toy **33** is shown in FIG. **3** in which a camouflage pattern **34** is employed. The camouflage pattern **34** may be any color, but since it is generally believed that many animals and most dogs are colorblind, it is the pattern rather than the colors used that are believed to be most important.

The camouflage pattern **34** helps to prevent location of the animal toy **10** by visual means. This requires the dog to locate the animal toy **10** by scent alone (such as when it is thrown).

The modified animal toy **33** includes a modified main segment **36** that is substantially curved. The curvature facilitates throwing, retrieval, and carrying of the modified animal toy **33**. It may also include the notch **13** (not shown in this drawing), as desired.

The invention has been shown, described, and illustrated in substantial detail with reference to the presently preferred embodiment. It will be understood by those skilled in this art that other and further changes and modifications may be made without departing from the spirit and scope of the invention which is defined by the claims appended hereto.

For example, the animal toy **10** may be used with other types of animals, other than dogs, to provide for either a dietary, chewing, or amusement benefit. Accordingly, the ingredients used to form the animal toy **10** are modified to optimally comply with the needs of whatever type of an animal is to use it.

What is claimed is:

1. An animal toy, comprising:

  (a) a solid main section having a diameter and a longitudinal length and extending a predetermined distance along said longitudinal length; and

  (b) at least one protrusion attached at one end thereof said main section and extending a predetermined distance therefrom and wherein said at least one protrusion includes a second longitudinal axis that is not in parallel alignment with a first longitudinal axis of said solid main section;

and wherein said animal toy is adapted to float on the water.

</td></tr>
</table>

US 6,360,693 B1

<table>
<tr><td align="center">5</td><td align="center">6</td></tr>
</table>

2. The animal toy of claim **1** wherein said main section is formed of a rubber.

3. The animal toy of claim **1** wherein said main section is formed of a plastic.

4. The animal toy of claim **1** wherein said main section includes a wood.

5. The animal toy of claim **1** wherein said main section includes cellulose.

6. The animal toy of claim **1** wherein said main section includes a flavoring.

7. The animal toy of claim **1** wherein said main section includes a scent added thereto.

8. The animal toy of claim **1** wherein said main section is rigid.

9. The animal toy of claim **1** wherein said main section is flexible.

10. The animal toy of claim **1** wherein said main section is chewable.

11. The animal toy of claim **1** wherein said main section includes a material that is lighter than water.

12. The animal toy of claim **1** wherein said animal toy includes a fluorescent coating.

13. The animal toy of claim **1** wherein said animal toy includes a camouflage coating.

14. The animal toy of claim **1** wherein said animal toy is formed of wood particles.

15. The animal toy of claim **1** wherein said animal toy is formed of wood chips.

16. The animal toy of claim **1** wherein said main section includes at least one notch, said at least one notch adapted to fracture said animal toy proximate said notch upon an application of sufficient lateral pressure to said animal toy.

17. A method for making an animal toy, which comprises:

compressing particles of cellulose together under pressure sufficient to retain said particles together when said pressure is removed so as to form said animal toy wherein said animal toy includes a main section having a first longitudinal axis and at least one protrusion extending therefrom and wherein said at least one protrusion includes a second longitudinal axis that is not parallel with respect to said first longitudinal axis and wherein said animal toy is adapted to float on the water.

18. The method of claim **17** including the step of adding a flavoring to said particles of cellulose prior to the step of compressing.

19. The method of claim **17** including the step of adding a resin to said particles of cellulose prior to the step of compressing.

20. The method of claim **17** wherein said particles are compressed so as to produce a main section having a diameter and a length and at least one protrusion attached thereto.

*   *   *   *   *

Appendix 5:
An Example of a National Institute of Health Biosketch

OMB No. 0925-0001 and 0925-0002 (Rev. 10/2021 Approved Through 01/31/2026)

BIOGRAPHICAL SKETCH

Provide the following information for the Senior/key personnel and other significant contributors.
Follow this format for each person. **DO NOT EXCEED FIVE PAGES.**

NAME: Gendreau, Julian

eRA COMMONS USER NAME (credential, e.g., agency login): GendreauJ

POSITION TITLE:

EDUCATION/TRAINING *(Begin with baccalaureate or other initial professional education, such as nursing, include postdoctoral training and residency training if applicable. Add/delete rows as necessary.)*

INSTITUTION AND LOCATION	DEGREE *(if applicable)*	Completion Date MM/YYYY	FIELD OF STUDY
University of Georgia	BS	05/2016	Microbiology
Mercer University School of Medicine	MD	05/2020	Medicine
Johns Hopkins University	MS	05/2024	Applied Biomedical Engineering

A. Personal Statement

My interest in the neurosciences began in medical school after learning about the interesting and complex nature of the human nervous system. In addition, it was in medical school that I learned of the many unknown aspects of the human nervous system and the great need for improvement of clinical care for these patients. Therefore, I began to have an interest in neurosurgery as it is one of the greatest fields where I can effectively advance the standard of care for patients in addition to providing the foremost optimal patient clinical care. During medical school, I began to gain clinical exposure of neurosurgery through my rotations and mentors. I also began to perform many clinical studies assessing patient outcomes of multiple different interventions.

B. Positions, Scientific Appointments, and Honors

Positions and Scientific Appointments

- Medical doctor, United States Army, 2021-2024
- PGY1 transitional year intern, Eisenhower Army Medical Center, 2020

Honors

- United States Army Health Professions Scholarship, United States Army, 2016
- Bachelor of Science with Highest Distinction, University of Georgia, 2016
- Phi Beta Kappa, University of Georgia, 2016
- Center for Undergraduate Research Assistantship Award, University of Georgia, 2015
- Plant Center Retreat, Best Undergraduate Research Award, University of Georgia, 2015
- Project Global Officer Fellowship for study in Morocco, United States Army, 2012

C.   Contributions to Science

Pre-doctoral
My pre-doctoral research mainly consists of clinical studies assessing patient outcomes after spinal and endovascular interventions in neurosurgery. This experience was key to enhancing my ability to retrieve data, perform statistical analysis, skillfully write manuscripts and submit manuscripts to journals for publication. I completed several projects with attendings across the United States before graduating medical school.

   a.   **Gendreau JL**, Kim LH, Prins PN, D'Souza M, Rezaii P, Pendharkar AV, Sussman ES, Ho AL, Desai AM. Outcomes After Cervical Disc Arthroplasty Versus Standalone Anterior Cervical Discectomy and Fusion: A Meta-analysis. Global Spine Journal 10(8): 1046-1056. December, 2020. PMID: 32875831.

   b.   Nathan JK, Foley J, Hoang T, Hiner J, Brooks S, **Gendreau JL**, Meurer WJ, Pandey AA, Adelman EE. The stroke navigator: meaningful use of the electronic health record to efficiently report inpatient stroke care quality. Journal of the American Medical Informatics Association 25(11): 1534-1539. November 1, 2018. PMID: 30124956.

   c.   D'Souza M, **Gendreau JL**, Feng A, Kim L, Ho AL, Veeravagu A. Robotic-assisted spine surgery: a review of itshistory, cost, and future trends. Robotic Surgery: Research and Reviews 6: 9-23. November 7, 2019. PMID: 31807602.

   d.   **Gendreau J**, Sheaffer K, Bennet J, Abraham M, Patel N, Herschman Y, Shaw E, Lindley J. Surgical intervention for dysphagia in patients with diffuse idiopathic skeletal hyperostosis: a meta-analysis. Clinical Spine Surgery 34(6):220-227. July 1, 2021. PMID: 33239502.

Post-Doctoral
My post-doctoral research includes many clinical outcomes studies in addition to device development. I began translating my clinical findings for creating novel devices. I have two submitted non-provisional patients for crowdsourced machine learning algorithms for both clinical providers and patients. I seek to continue this translational ability with application to incorporating patient imaging into clinical outcomes studies.

Peer-Reviewed Manuscripts
   a.   **Gendreau J**, Jimenez A, Kuo C, Lozinsky S, Zenonos G, Gardner P, Raza S, Dea N, Gokaslan Z, Choby G, Van Gompel J, Redmond K, Gallia G, Bettegowda C, Rowan N, Kuo C, Mukherjee D. Radiotherapy after Gross Total Resection of Skull Base Chordoma: A Survival and Epidemiological and End Results Database Analysis of Survival Outcomes. World Neurosurgery. November 12, 2022.

   b.   **Gendreau J**, Kuo C, Mehkri Y, Chakravarti S, Lu B, Lubelski D, Redmond K, Bettegowda C, Mukherjee D. Radiotherapy after gross total resection and subtotal resection of spinal chordoma: A SEER database analysis of overall survival outcomes. Journal of Neurosurgery Spine. March 7, 2023.

   c.   **Gendreau J**, Mehkri Y, Kuo C, Chakravarti S, Jimenez M, Shalom M, Kazemi F, Mukherjee D. Clinical Predictors of Overall Survival in Very Elderly Glioblastoma Patients: A National Cancer Database Analysis. Neurosurgery. Accepted March 10, 2024.

   d.   **Gendreau J**, Gowda K, Kazemi F, Horowitz M, Shalom M, Kuo C, Mehkri Y, Yan M, Redmond K, Lubelski D, Mukherjee D. Fractionated radiotherapy after gross total resection of spinal chordoma: A systematic review of survival outcomes using individualized patient data. Journal of Neurosurgery: Spine. Accepted June 7, 2024.

Please find a complete listing of my peer-reviewed work at:
https://www.ncbi.nlm.nih.gov/myncbi/1tAaTKEmcczQG/bibliography/public/

Appendix 6:
An Example of a National Institutes of Health "Other Support" Document

OTHER SUPPORT

Gendreau, Julian
Commons ID: GendreauJ

<u>ACTIVE</u>

None.

PENDING

None.

Overlap

None.

IN KIND

None.

I, PD/PI or other senior/key personnel, certify that the statements herein are true, complete and accurate to the best of my knowledge, and accept the obligation to comply with Public Health Services terms and conditions if a grant is awarded as a result of this application. I am aware that any false, fictitious, or fraudulent statements or claims may subject me to criminal, civil, or administrative penalties.

*Signature:
Date: _____________________

Index